SKIN SOBERING

skin
SOBERING

99% OF PRODUCTS AGE AND HARM YOUR SKIN

LEARN WHAT YOU TRULY NEED TO BE BEAUTIFUL AND MAKEUP-READY

ERIN YUET TJAM, PHD
& RYUICHI UTSUGI, MD

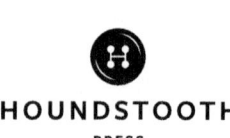

HOUNDSTOOTH
PRESS

COPYRIGHT © 2023 ERIN YUET TJAM
All rights reserved.

SKIN SOBERING
99% of Products Age and Harm Your Skin:
Learn What You Truly Need to Be Beautiful and Makeup-Ready

ISBN 978-1-5445-3887-7 *Hardcover*
      978-1-5445-3888-4 *Paperback*
      978-1-5445-3889-1 *Ebook*
      978-1-5445-3950-8 *Audiobook*

For my Baba. I wish I had known better so you could have left us feeling comfortable and not itchy. Beauty and health were my motivation to practice Skin Sobering, but you were my fuel to write this book.

contents

Preface **ix**
Introduction **xiii**

1. REALIZATION 1
What Started and Sustained the Skincare Product Craze

2. EVIDENCE 23
What Scientists and Doctors (Who Don't Sell Products) Say about Our Skin

3. DISBELIEF 51
We've Been Lied To

4. (BIO)CHEMISTRY 67
Products That Claim to Heal Us Are Hurting Us

5. DAMAGE 83
How Does Our Body Incur and Respond to Damage?

6. EPIDEMIC 89
Skin Problems and Diseases Are at All-Time Highs

7. PROBLEMS 97
How Do We Handle Our Skin When We Love It and Hate It?

8. GUIDE 129
How to Be Simply Beautiful with Skin Sobering

9. PRODUCTS 165
...and Promises with No Proof

10. LIFESTYLE 181
How You Live Affects How You Look

11. CONFUSION 209
Constant Celebrity Endorsements Make Us Trust Products

12. HEALTH 221
...Is How We Get to Beauty

13. CHANGE 241
Drop the Marketing Nonsense and Adopt New Behaviors Based on Science

14. MY STORY 257

15. YOUR WAY 267
Skincare Products Are like Drugs, Treats, and Makeup—Don't Use Them Every Day

Conclusion 279
The End...of All the Secrets! 283
Acknowledgments 291
Appendix for Chinese Sayings 295
Notes 299
About the Authors 311
Professional Achievements 317

preface

Skin Sobering seems completely at odds with today's skin care theories and marketing. It isn't surprising when people react with a combination of disbelief, doubt, and resistance. Unlike the skin of so many people seeking help and answers, the science in this case is clear.

We are ex-product worshipper, Beauty-Obsessed Scientist Erin Yuet Tjam, PhD, and renowned physician in anti-aging, board-certified plastic surgeon, and skin health and beauty author, Ryuichi Utsugi, MD. Together, we have 70 years of experience in the medical, health, and skin care industries.

Dr. Tjam is a bicultural, bilingual health scientist and an adjunct professor whose work has been published in numerous peer-reviewed journals. Over the course of her career, Dr. Tjam has been awarded over $7.5 million in research grants. In 2009, she was appointed by David Johnston as his special advisor when he was President of the University of Waterloo (he later became the Governor General of Canada). Dr. Tjam also holds honorary professorships at several universities in China. Prior to learning about Dr. Utsugi's work, Dr. Tjam did many things to her skin in the name of vanity. For nearly 40 years, she tried all kinds of increasingly expensive "lotions and potions," as well as certain in-clinic treatments. These serums, creams, and moisturizers didn't resolve any of the problems for which they were marketed. When the products were on Erin's skin, they appeared to produce desirable effects, but as soon as the products were off, all her skin problems reappeared. In fact, many of them had gotten worse.

Dr. Utsugi is a highly respected reconstructive burn specialist and plastic surgeon with over four decades of work experience. He has made significant contributions to the field. Early in his career, Dr. Utsugi regularly recommended skincare products to patients and even planned to mass produce his own line once he retired from clinical practice. However, while working as an expert advisor to several skincare companies, Dr. Utsugi discovered skincare products were not delivering on their promises. Instead, he discovered they slowly worsen and damage the skin. He has presented this groundbreaking research at over 160 conferences, published 19 scientific papers, produced 13 medical textbooks, and 7 skin health books. One of his books, 「肌」の悩みがすべて消えるたった1つの方法　美肌には化粧水もクリームもいりません[1] (*The Only Way to Get Rid of All Your Skin Problems. You Don't Need Lotion or Cream for Beautiful Skin.*) was translated into four languages and is sold across Asia. This revolutionary book popularized the idea of discontinuing the use of skincare products as a means to clean, nourish, and beautify your skin.

In short, Dr. Utsugi once sold and recommended skincare products, and Dr. Tjam once used them! Today, we have joined forces to share the most crucial thing we've discovered over the course of our lives and careers: almost every product out there produces long-lasting harm to your skin, even when those products make it look or feel better—*temporarily*. There is compelling and indisputable evidence behind why you should quit using skincare products, and our goal is to share that information with as many people as possible.

Dr. Utsugi has been advocating the *Skin Sobering* skin care method for over 20 years, and for good reason. It is evident that the persistent practice of the good habits outlined in this book can resolve almost every skin beauty problem. Of course, there are a couple of conditions even *Skin Sobering* cannot correct, but those afflicted individuals will still find the information offered here beneficial.

Skin Sobering is an uncomplicated skin care method that not only heals your skin, it simplifies your life and frees your spirit. In fact, *Skin Sobering* is so straightforward and simple, you can accurately claim it is organic, natural, locally obtained, ethically sourced, non-GMO, free of animal cruelty, environmentally conscious, socially responsible, politically correct, gender neutral, wallet friendly, time-saving, and life-simplifying—all the same buzz phrases and lofty appeals skincare companies have tried to claim and have fallen short on delivering. In line with Dr. Utsugi's research, you will find *Skin Sobering* meets all these high standards and makes your skin more beautiful and healthy.

In its simplest form, *Skin Sobering* is the scientifically proven, research-backed advice to just stop using products and care for your skin with water.

It really is that simple. So why are we dedicating a whole book to explaining it? Well, to quit smoking, "all" you have to do is not smoke. To abstain from alcohol, "just" stop drinking. If you want to be fit, "simply" start moving. To diet, it's "easy": eat less and avoid junk food.

The point is, the solution may sound simple but it is often easier said than done.

It is the same for *Skin Sobering*. The action itself is very simple, but learning how to do it or why anyone should even bother is a lot more complicated. What should you do when you run into problems? How do you recognize what is a problem and what is just a phase? What should you do when you are weak, when you want to give up, when you doubt the method, and when you doubt yourself? This book exists to help you answer these questions.

Skin Sobering is not just a discussion of Dr. Utsugi's discoveries and his life's work. Dr. Tjam also provides support for his clinical proof and shows you the scientific studies, historical evidence, legal matters, industry strategies, celebrity tales, and more, that expose skincare products don't just affect skin beauty—they are tightly linked with skin sensitivity and diseases. These conditions have reached epidemic proportions in children and older adults.

It's time to discard your old beliefs—the ones the skincare industry and its partners have spent billions of dollars marketing to you. We will reveal the loopholes and strategies these companies are using to claim their products are wonderful. Most of all, we will teach you how to care for your skin with a simple approach that actually works.

It is our hope that armed with the information shared in this book, you will feel motivated to stop using products that damage and halt regeneration of your skin. We want to empower you by sharing what we know, so you can make informed choices moving forward. We hope you will feel, as we both do, energized and happy to share your success with your loved ones so they too can benefit.

We wish you joy and beauty!

introduction

FROM THE BEAUTY-OBSESSED SCIENTIST, ERIN YUET TJAM, PHD

Many people know I'm a health scientist, but very few know I'm also a die-hard "girly girl" obsessed with having great-looking skin. Or maybe I have that backward. I didn't stop using skincare products for environmental, financial, time-saving, or health reasons. Those may be better motivations to practice *Skin Sobering*, but my motivation was purely beauty. Writing this book, on the other hand, was driven by an entirely different purpose.

My school friends of over 40 years and I make every effort to meet annually in Hong Kong. We eat and talk about life, health, and beauty. During one of our annual meet-ups, the prettiest one, Jackie, mentioned a bestselling Japanese book with a Chinese title, *Skin Fasting*, written by a physician named Ryuichi Utsugi 宇津木龍一.[2] This book was on the bestseller list for five years in Japan. It was translated into four languages and published in China, Korea, Thailand, Hong Kong, Taiwan, and Macau. *Skin Fasting* chronicled thousands of clinical cases, sharing evidence that revealed skincare products weren't working as advertised, as well as the science behind skin physiology and product chemistry. It revealed why skincare products—to my horror, even cleansers!—are some of the biggest culprits of skin problems, beaten only by UV rays and poor lifestyle choices.

At the time, I'd been living like beauty always came first. If something made my skin healthier but not more visibly beautiful right away, I wouldn't listen. I was a diligent skincare user and skillful makeup gal, so I looked quite good when the products were on. But when I cleaned them off my face, my skin was dry and looked a shade of dull, yellowish-gray.

I couldn't believe skin "care" products could harm my skin. I did know makeup wasn't all wonderful. I didn't want to agree with what I was learning because I had trusted skincare products most of my life—and I am smart, damn it! Yet my skin issues had only worsened over the years, despite all my diligent skin care routines. I had clogged pores, blackheads, fine lines, dark under-eye circles, puffy eyes, hyperpigmentation, dullness, uneven tone, thin skin, bumps, dryness, dehydration, sensitivity, inflammation, breakouts…Waah! It was awful!

I was resourceful and skillful *and* vain, so I learned to cover all these flaws with "natural-looking" makeup before I faced the world each day. Thanks to my efforts, very few friends noticed my skin issues, and, of course, none of them knew how much time I had to spend to hide them.

By age 53, I was exhausted with these morning and evening routines of putting on and taking off my face. My lovely husband was patient every night, and my dear kids were tolerant every time we were to go out, but *I* was fed up. I wanted so badly to look good, but my method was just not working. My skin wasn't looking better in spite of all the labor I put into its upkeep. Now that I had lived over half a century, my skin and I had finally experienced enough to see past the marketing of "miracle" skin solutions I so desperately wished were true.

After digesting Dr. Utsugi's book, the science *finally* got through to me—and I'm a health scientist! Can you believe the power of marketing? Skin is not meant to be "nourished" with products, and it's not meant to absorb them either. It is an *excretory organ* meant to *eliminate waste*!

Before my 30s, my skin used to bounce back no matter what I did to it. We all feel invincible at younger ages, taking one risk after another. Now I know what I took for granted as "invincibility" just translated to invisible damage that accumulated over time. One day, that damage surfaces, and it isn't concealable. For me, it happened in my mid-40s. I needed to do the right thing immediately if I wanted my skin to look beautiful.

I quit skincare products. The withdrawal phase of quitting felt like what people describe when they give up smoking. Improvement was gradual but noticeable. It took me three months, but my skin was revived! Thank goodness not consuming skincare products also helps the environment, saves money and time, simplifies life, and results in healthier skin. Of course, doing the right thing also gave me the prize I really wanted: not just healthy, but beautiful skin.

I felt so indebted to Dr. Utsugi for "saving my skin" that I tracked him down and built up the courage to send him a heartfelt letter of gratitude. He wrote back! Not only did I get to exchange with him, but I even convinced him to write this new book in English together!

We decided that because skincare products are not nutrients, the process of ending their use is not really like fasting. When fasting, a person stops eating for a while but eventually eats again. Instead, we wanted to describe quitting something your body doesn't need though you've come to depend on its temporarily desirable effects. That is a sobering process, and thus *Skin Sobering* was born.

FROM THE ANTI-AGING DOCTOR, RYUICHI UTSUGI 宇津木龍一, MD

Beauty-conscious women have more skin problems.

This is a bold statement, but it is backed by clinical research and the scientific community. Surveys show that more than 80% of Japanese women have dry skin,[3] and 40–60% have sensitive skin.[4] Why do so many women have skin problems? There are lots of reasons, but I believe the main one is they are reliant on skincare products.

In 1999, I founded the Aesthetic Medicine Center of the Research Institute of Kitasato University Hospital in Tokyo (北里大学北里研究所病院, 形成外科, 美容外科), where I performed skin examinations for outpatients. It was quite a hit. Many women who pay attention to skin care came to get their skin analyzed—although they didn't think they had many skin issues.

We assessed their skin with a handheld microscope. To my surprise and theirs, more than 80% of them had severely dry skin and inflamed pores. Even more surprising, when they stopped using skincare products, the dehydration, dryness, and inflammation significantly improved, along with other seemingly unrelated problems. As soon as they resumed using the products, their skin conditions worsened again.

Upon examining these skincare products, we found that all of them contained surfactants, preservatives, fragrances, and/or oils. These substances affect the skin's natural abilities to protect and repair itself. It's been well-documented in scientific literature that the best way to take care of our skin is to protect it, to *not* interfere with its natural functioning, and to *not* use any products—cleansers, makeup removers, toners, serums, masks, moisturizers, lotions, creams, and more inventive names we can't keep up with. And natural or organic products are *all* processed, making them not much different from their synthetic counterparts, just more expensive. Put simply, *sober up* your skin and allow it to repair, rejuvenate, and restore its beauty. This is what your skin needs. Most skin beauty problems (and many diseases) are caused by products altering the skin's protective and regenerative functions.

Skin care is medically grouped under dermatology, but my skin care concept and practice came from burn care—an approach based on healing theory. When I was a reconstructive plastic surgeon at the teaching hospital, I specialized in the treatment of severe burns. The most important aspect of treating burns is to not let the skin get dry. If burned skin gets dry, it can die, and so can the patient. So, during the process of treating burns, the goal is to help the skin stay hydrated and to regenerate. Using oil-based lotions or creams to keep skin moist is a definite *no-no*. They will damage the skin, which is common medical knowledge. These products are foreign substances to vulnerable, defenseless, and injured skin. They are essentially toxins to the skin. The skin will reject these foreign agents by inflaming, forming pus, and not being able to grow new cells.

When you apply skincare products to healthy skin, their effect is not so severe as to cause the skin to form pus, but they will weaken the skin's protective barrier and regenerative abilities. Moisture will escape, and the skin will become dehydrated. When products get into the pores, the skin silently gets irritated and inflamed—the catalyst for many other skin problems. Dryness, sensitivity, puffiness, fine lines, and a long list of skin conditions typically associated with aging are all essentially symptoms of a common root problem: skincare products, both synthetic and natural. This includes cleansers. The women who came to get their skin analyzed appeared to have different skin issues, but all of them stemmed from the same underlying causes: interferences to their skin's innate metabolisms.

Even though I am now considered an expert on the negative effects of skincare products, and I am a strong advocate for simple ways to care for the skin, I used to be like many cosmetic doctors who recommended and sold skincare products. I am not only a reconstructive and burn specialist, I am a plastic surgeon and was an expert advisor to skincare companies. Because of these experiences and relationships, I spent a lot of time on skin care research and planned to establish my own skincare company after I retired from my clinical practice. That was when I truly believed skincare products offered nutrients to the skin and helped our skin to be beautiful (like many other doctors who sell skincare products). That is, I believed this until I discovered the opposite.

Back in 1997, I was not an expert in skin care yet. So, I read all the books on skin I could find, and I consulted with my dermatologist colleagues on how to care for the skin. The consensus among them was that the three most important things for skin health and beauty were protection, proper cleansing, and preserving the skin's moisture. This was what dermatology textbooks have said all along, and it felt achievable in my mind. I was excited and ambitious, so I embarked on developing a skincare line for my patients that was safe and effective. I used the best ingredients and no preservatives. When someone experienced an undesirable reaction, I tested each of the ingredients to find the irritant. I even customized products by removing ingredients that triggered someone's allergic reaction. I also developed an allergy strip to aid the new product line. I called it "allergy-tested skin care."

This line included five fundamental skincare products: cleanser, toner, lotion and cream, oil, and sunscreen. They were very popular among my patients and were highly sought after. In the 1990s, cosmeceuticals (medical cosmetics) were just becoming popular, and cosmetics companies were after me to market these products. I was encouraged and quite excited to develop a commercial line for the general market. I hired a renowned designer for the package design and chose syringe-style tubes as containers so the product content would stay airtight during use.

This allergy-tested skincare line went through vigorous research and endless testing but, in the end, I chose not to launch it to the general public. I stopped my products from being mass distributed, and I personally quit using all products.

Why?

Because I discovered that skincare products, including my meticulously formulated, "irritation-free" ones, cause the skin to be inflamed and dry. They also eventually decrease the skin's innate metabolic functioning. Essentially, the more products a person uses, the worse his or her skin condition becomes. And it isn't *just* the preservatives and allergens in the products, as we had initially thought.

So, to my English readers around the world, whether your skin is beautiful or not has a lot to do with genetics and lifestyle, but also what you put your skin through. It has nothing to do with nationality or "race." *Skin Sobering* is an effective method suitable for all skin types—for all people—to bring their skin to its best shape. This is based on more than 20 years of clinical practice and an evidence-based skin care "secret formula." To call it a secret is an exaggeration. It is really a simple formula of not disrupting your skin and cleaning it purposefully and diligently with water. Your skin will restore its optimal functioning. Persistence is the hard part, like all good habits in life, and you may need time and knowledge to be convinced to change. Even though *Skin Sobering* is beneficial and great for all skin, not everyone can start *Skin Sobering* at full tilt because people have different degrees of skin damage and product dependency. That alone is the clearest evidence that the world needs *Skin Sobering*.

Thousands of my patients who now practice *Skin Sobering* all report the same experience:

"Everyone says my skin looks much better."

"My skin feels so good!"

"I am not spending time and money on skincare products, and my skin is beautiful."

"There are no more bottles and containers! My makeup counter and my skin have both cleared up!"

We know why skincare products damage the skin. We know the best way to care for the skin. And we know how people can achieve the healthiest and most beautiful skin. The dissemination of these answers is my new, ambitious plan.

FROM THE BEAUTY-OBSESSED SCIENTIST

BEAUTY, PUBLIC HEALTH, AND SCIENCE

BEAUTY...

I practice *Skin Sobering* for its beauty benefits. All the other excellent reasons really don't matter much if my skin is not becoming more beautiful. You may very well practice *Skin Sobering* for all the right reasons, and kudos to you, sincerely! But I'm admittedly vain. So while the environment, your health, and your pocketbook benefit from quitting skincare products, I practice *Skin Sobering* because it makes my skin more beautiful, and it will make yours more beautiful too.

There's nothing wrong with wanting to be beautiful. Beauty has been described as an emotional response and as a feeling you just know. Beauty, while cultural and subjective, makes us feel good—beauty in animals, in nature, in art, and architecture, in what we create, and in what we see within ourselves. It's a hard thing to define, but we know it when we see it, and we want it.

There may not be a universal standard for beauty, but there is one for health and healthy skin. Healthy skin is skin that can maintain its natural beauty, which is *not* the same as flawless skin—natural beauty has flaws. And, like a healthy body, healthy skin has the ability to fight injuries and diseases quickly and effectively.

This all comes down to a strong barrier function—the most important function of the skin. We are surrounded by germs, pollutants, irritants, contaminants, toxins, and UV radiation. When our skin has a strong barrier function, it can resist these insults and heal quickly. It can also generate plumper skin by retaining water and reducing moisture loss.[5] A weak barrier function, on the other hand, will experience more intense aggravation, take longer to recover, and will not completely restore to its original state, thereby leaving marks, spots, dips, lumps, lines, and scars—that is unhealthy skin, and it's not pretty. Skincare products slowly but surely weaken this barrier.

To visually *recognize* healthy skin is not as tricky as judging beauty, and the lines between them do cross. Healthy skin looks bright, supple, smooth, clear, soft, and intact. It is neither dry, flaky, nor inflamed.

In essence, healthy skin looks naturally beautiful.

A PUBLIC HEALTH MISSION...

Is beauty really that important? Beautiful things attract our eyes, but who defines what is beautiful? Do we only celebrate beauty and ignore inner character? Is beauty confused with worth? These are philosophical and social questions that I am not able to address adequately in this book, but I recognize their importance. So why am I waving the "beauty flag" and labeling myself a beauty-obsessed scientist knowing the complexity of this construct? Am I talking out of both sides of my mouth?

Yes, I am! I have a bigger purpose: a public health mission. Doctors and scientists can talk till their faces turn blue about health matters, yet they are unable to attract the attention of the general public. After all, beauty attracts and beauty sells. So, we will wave the beauty flag first to bait your attention. Then we will show you the deeper meaning of *Skin Sobering*—to stop the hidden epidemic of skin problems that affect you, your children, and your elderly parents.

This is not a shallow, skin-deep issue.

Skin diseases *are* an epidemic. The prevalence of childhood eczema—a common first sign for a group of conditions known as the "atopic march"[6] (including hay fever, asthma, and food allergies)—is skyrocketing. These are not skin-deep matters. Nor are cystic acne, dermatitis, or psoriasis, which are recognized skin diseases that are starting earlier in life and lasting longer.

Then there are conditions like sensitivity, dryness, and itchiness, all of which are often dismissed as shallow or *normal* skin annoyances. Yet the rate of these problems is rising steeply,[7] especially in young and vulnerable populations like babies and the frail elderly[8,9]—individuals who are cared for by others, who don't have the choice to use or not use products. The prevalence of these irritating conditions doesn't even compare to the rampant beauty issues of dehydration, fine lines, uneven tone, dullness, puffiness, hyperpigmentation, wrinkles, sagginess, and so on. Clinicians have known for a long time that minor, superficial issues, and severe skin conditions are worsened by products, so ironically, many issues are self-induced. But, the majority of product users don't suspect any correlation between the skincare products they use and their existing or worsening skin problems.[10] Why would they? The products they're buying are marketed as "skin saviors," so why would the end user believe they're doing more harm than good? Makeup may be a suspect, but skin "care" products?

When you know something is bad for you and you choose to indulge cautiously (e.g., junk food, alcohol, sugar), that's one thing. When you've been misinformed and kept in the dark all your life, that's a whole different story. The truth needs to be told. If we can draw your attention to skin health in any way, even *through* beauty, we will. *Skin Sobering* links two concepts that need to be linked: a rampant public health issue and skin beauty.

WHAT WE KNOW ALREADY...

Skincare products are not the worst thing for your skin. They are just one of the bad things, along with UV rays, smoking, and a bad lifestyle. I knew about sun, smoke, and sugar, but I didn't have a clue that skincare products were also harming my skin. I didn't want to believe it even once I became aware of it. I had not done any of the other bad things, so I know now that my skin was not in its top beauty form because of my genes and fastidious use of skincare products.

Skin issues are deemed shallow and superficial because that is where this organ lies on our body. Yes, your skin is in fact an organ. Skin issues can seem minor when compared to problems experienced by other organs. The skin, at its worst, will be scaly and inflamed, but usually it is just itchy, dry, or sensitive—issues not even significant enough to be classified as medical symptoms. What compounds this is many people feel that product users *eat their own bad fruit* 自食其果 (zi shi qi guo)—they are getting a taste of their own medicine. Or worse, they brought the issues on themselves 自作自受 (zi zuo zi shou)—*self-inflicted, so it serves you right*. These users are believed to fuss too much over their skin and indulge in products, so they are dismissed as vain. These judgments mostly apply to women who use makeup products.

It seems like deep down, a lot of people already know that some products are not good for their skin. However, the pervasive nature of decades of nonstop advertising and misinformation have created massive cognitive dissonance for consumers. Physicians and scientists know that *makeup* products harm our skin, regardless of how pure, natural, or organic the formulations claim to be. They are all chemicals. So, when women report problems with their skin but continue to use makeup, it's predictable that both physicians and regular folks feel compelled to privately roll their eyes. How bad could it really be if you continue to contribute to your own problem, just for looks?

This "you-deserve-it" judgment has some degree of truth to it. However, what is not known to all these diligent customers (including physicians!) is that it is not *just* makeup that affects the skin. It's skincare products as well, including cleansers. Unfortunately, people use skincare products because they have been led to believe these products provide nutrients to the skin. That's the reason they do it. The reality is, skincare products are essentially colorless makeup products. The majority of consumers have no idea that the gentle cleansers, organic lotions, and award-winning creams and serums that claim to protect and repair skin are the cause of skin sensitivity and other problems.

To be clear, you do need to clean and protect your skin—just not with skincare products.

Skincare products will worsen your skin's functionality and restorative abilities, despite their ability to temporarily make your skin appear to improve. Skincare products at best should be treated like makeup, used for occasional enhancement and with the understanding that those temporary enhancements come with a more long-term price.

Skin problems became more prevalent as our society became more "civilized" and more products were being promoted. Now, this is no longer a superficial women-deserve-these-problems-because-they-bring-them-on-themselves situation, but a lack of knowledge and falling victim to powerful marketing (of misinformation). The fact is, most people have no idea that skincare products are actually harming their skin, despite giving their skin some short-lived visual effects, which we've been taught to crave. These effects disappear once the product does, leaving skin issues in their wake.

SCIENCE...

Why has science and nature lost the battle to convince you that when you cleanse your skin with face wash or make this excretory organ absorb lotion, you are acting against nature? Why is it that when your skin fights back with signs of dryness, oiliness, puffiness, pigmentation, acne, sensitivity, itchiness, dullness, clogged pores, blemishes, bumps, or breakouts, you attribute these signs to your skin misbehaving and assume it is in need of more products?

Because marketing is way louder than science, in spite of all science's evidence. You've probably never had a chance to *ignore* the science, because you've never heard it in the first place; the beauty industry and its excessive marketing have drowned it out.

The beauty industry spends mega bucks ($11.5 billion *a year, a company*, on marketing,[11] to be precise) to buy endorsements from professionals and megastars to influence your grandma, your mom, and you. If that is not convincing enough, those who have already drunk the Kool-Aid are people we love and want to listen to—Jennifer, Angelina, Ellen, Sofia, Helen, Kari, Tessa, Gwyneth...Gosh, this is an impossible battle!

So, how are we going to address your doubts, misconceptions, and a lifelong practice bolstered by generations of tradition? Through basic science, epidemiology, unencumbered physicians' words, personal testimonials, and celebrity stories, and by exposing the strategies of the beauty industry, the power of the advertising world, the ambiguities of the legal system, and the temptations from your digital and real surroundings.

If we are able to exert any influence, we will upset the beauty industry and threaten the livelihood of many professionals—aestheticians, cosmetologists, makeup artists, spa owners, beauty editors, bloggers, retailers, importers, exporters, manufacturers, school owners, marketing specialists, researchers, nurses, doctors, surgeons, and my friend Jolanta who owns a spa—like the smoking cessation movement that angered the tobacco world. Skincare products are not half as bad as tobacco, but they also don't do 1/100th of the good that you believe!

We hope that when you practice *Skin Sobering* and see results, you will give us a shout-out. Marketing is unfortunately way louder than science, so we need your help to make some noise. Thanks to decades of misinformation, it's no small feat to back a method that whispers of a simpler life and healthier, more beautiful skin.

1
REALIZATION
WHAT STARTED AND SUSTAINED THE SKINCARE PRODUCT CRAZE

SOAP OPERAS—HOW THE MARKETING MANIPULATION BEGAN

CLEANLINESS VS. HYGIENE

GERMS VS. IMMUNE SYSTEM

PROMOTE. PROMOTE. PROMOTE.

THE LEGAL VACUUM

FROM THE BEAUTY-OBSESSED SCIENTIST

SOAP OPERAS—HOW THE MARKETING MANIPULATION BEGAN

Whatever age you are, you have probably been using skincare products for about that long. In fact, most people in the developed world have been using skincare products almost from birth. Well-intentioned moms wash their babies with sweetly scented infant products from the get-go—I did this with all my babies. Anytime my firstborn got something on his skin, I would clean it with a soap or a body wash right away, followed by a moisturizer to soothe his skin.

Thankfully, my third son didn't get that attention—I was too worn out! The idea that your skin is not clean unless it is washed with a chemical, and the belief that your skin will not be beautiful unless you care for it with products are socially ingrained in us, and amplified since the "Soap Opera Era" of the 1940s.

Dr. Sandy Skotnicki, a well-known dermatologist in Toronto, said in her book *Beyond Soap*, "Our obsessive washing today has more to do with the advertising industry's ability to play on our insecurities than any health-related need to ensure the hygiene of the skin."[12]

Starting in the early years of the 20th century, the soap industry was one of America's largest advertisers, according to Harvard business historian Dr. Geoffrey Jones.[13] Our hygienic behavior has evolved from the germ theory to the hygiene hypothesis and is now best described as a cleanliness *obsession*. Jones also wrote that the advent of soap and washing was a symbol of social status and the moral superiority of Western civilization. Soap was not just advertised as a tool for human cleanliness; it was the first widely available *beauty product*. Soap itself was a statement—it needed to be used to make one acceptable to polite society. Human odors became shameful and distasteful. Jones noted that in many advertisements, "The right soaps promised to signal social respectability, and even to transform one's romantic life."

The North American soap market continued to grow throughout post-WWII to include cleansers, beauty bars, balms, and moisturizers. All were designed to "cure" our insecurities, even though many of those insecurities came from advertising delivered by the soap companies to begin with. It is therefore not difficult to see that our initial desire to be hygienic and healthy very quickly morphed into a full-blown cultural obsession that has little to do with health or hygiene. Instead, it has created an epidemic of skin problems.

How did the soap industry's influence reach so wide and deep? To help them sell, these early skin care companies created an entire new class of entertainment—soap operas—to sell cleansers and detergents. It started in the 1930s when one company sponsored each show and controlled all the ads. Procter & Gamble (P&G) sponsored a number of early radio dramas and was soon followed by similar industry leaders like Colgate-Palmolive and Lever Brothers (now Unilever). The ensuing radio and daytime TV shows were purposely used as a vehicle to advertise soaps and detergents to housewives. *Painted Dreams, Ma Perkins, The Guiding Light, The Archers, Coronation Street, General Hospital, Days of Our Lives, The Young and the Restless, As the World Turns*—some of these are still running today. They have been incredibly successful for over 80 years and are deeply rooted in Western culture just like the products they promote.

We have been programmed to believe cleaning requires chemicals. In fact, the phrase "spic and span" references a brand of all-purpose household cleaner introduced in the 1930s of the same name. By the 1940s, P&G had made Spic and Span famous by constantly advertising it during soap operas. As a result, the brand not only became imprinted in consumer memory, it became *the* metaphor for something looking clean and spotless.

My mom cleans her kitchen three times a day, but she rarely uses detergents, so her kitchen always smells like food. Unlike my mother, I spent my formative years in the Western world at the mercy of advertising, so I wanted my kitchen to smell lemony fresh. I used scented detergents the moment something came into contact with grease, as if grease was my sworn enemy to be defeated only by artificial freshness. I have friends who wash their dishes in soapy water, then leave them on the drying rack, or dry them with tea towels—no rinsing. They like the scent the soap product leaves on their dishes. Others use shine products in their dishwasher cycle so their dishes come out sparkling—not just clean, but literally *sparkling* with chemicals. Some friends will have a bubble bath and pat themselves dry afterward without rinsing.

To them and to so many more people, chemicals mean *clean*.

CLEANLINESS VS. HYGIENE

When patients go to a doctor's office with a skin problem, the first thing they say is often, "I've been cleaning it!"[14] People wash so much because they believe it makes them civilized, keeps them healthy, and that makes them feel more beautiful. This fixation on cleanliness is promoted everywhere. From bleaching and sanitizing your house, to removing 99.9% of germs on your hands. We do this in the name of protecting our family or to prevent some other dire situation.

Is the fear of germs and dirt keeping our skin and body healthy, or is it contributing to the epidemic of skin problems? Are germs really so frightening?

To answer this, we need to understand hygiene versus cleanliness.[15] They are different. Hygiene involves practices to protect us from *infectious diseases*. Washing your hands after you cough or sneeze, use the bathroom, ride public transport, or touch railings and surfaces in public spaces is a smart, hygienic practice. You are removing potentially harmful germs you may have come in contact with.

Cleanliness, on the other hand, is more socially defined. To be "clean," we must be free of all dirt, all germs, feel fresh, and have either no smell or, better yet, smell of freshly scented cleansers, lotions, and sprays. This sort of cleanliness is highly cultural and is about a desire for social acceptability—not what is best for our skin or health. The washing practices that keep us healthy and *hygienic* differ from the washing process we've been socialized into believing make us *clean*. The frequency, vigor, and amount of chemicals we use to stay clean far exceed hygienic requirements. We wash our body, hair, and face so much that we're damaging our skin's protective barrier, making us much more prone to disease. We are exposing our skin to products that are harming what we want to protect.[16]

It is only in the last 80 years that cleaning and grooming have become daily customs, and this timeline coincides exactly with the rising epidemic of skin problems. Before the 1940s, in our millions of years of existence, humans did not clean once, twice, or three times a day with soaps, cleansers, and chemicals. Now, millions of people around the world are stuck in a cycle of skin damage: drying their skin with cleansers, temporarily fixing this dryness with lotions and creams, then concealing the resulting problems with makeup. With each layer added, more cleansers are needed, causing further dryness, dehydration, and damage. We put our skin through an endless cycle of damage and concealment, reinforcing an existing problem by hiding it, worsening it, and ultimately wrecking it.

GERMS VS. IMMUNE SYSTEM

The debate of germs, hygiene, cleanliness, and the body started well before the 1940s. When COVID-19 hit, the 150-year-old controversy of germ theory versus terrain theory resurfaced. Karen Selick wrote an OP-ED, stating:

> Louis Pasteur (1822–1895) the father of germ theory popularized the idea that we become sick when our bodies are invaded by foreign organisms such as bacteria, molds, fungi, and viruses. What's not widely known is that other French scientists Antoine Béchamp (1816–1908) and Claude Bernard (1813–1878), had somewhat different beliefs, known as the terrain theory. They believed that the most important factor that determines whether or not a person becomes ill is *not* the presence of germs, but rather the preparedness of the body's internal environment (the "soil" or terrain), to repel or destroy the germs.[17]

Essentially, terrain theory ensures the immune system is operating at peak efficiency to mount a successful defense. The reputation of Pasteur versus Béchamp was quite similar to that of Thomas Edison versus Nikola Tesla. For financial, largely unscientific reasons, Pasteur and Edison crushed Béchamp and Tesla, respectively.

Germs are everywhere; they are a permanent, vast, and unavoidable part of our world. Most of them exist inside and on our body in a symbiotic relationship. Béchamp reported that it was only when the cells of the host became damaged or compromised that germs could manifest as a prevailing *symptom* (not a cause) of disease. Despite their bitter war when they were living, at the end of Pasteur's life, he reportedly recognized the importance of what Béchamp had been trying to tell him, remarking, "*Béchamp avait raison. Le germ n'est rien, c'est le terrain qui est tout.*" Béchamp was right. The germ is nothing, it's the soil that is everything.[18] And the world now praises and thanks Tesla's alternating current (AC) invention almost as much as Edison's direct current (DC).

Germ versus terrain theory is still a point of contention among scientists, journalists, and us plebeians. However, germ theory has won over medical schools and the healthcare industry. Since the last century, medical teaching has largely been about preventing germs from infecting the body. This idea has become foundational for medical professionals for the past 150 years. There is no doubt that humans benefited from reduced exposure to pathogens. Scientists developed antibiotics to fight off bacterial infections so mortality rates caused by infectious diseases, such as cholera, typhoid, tuberculosis, dysentery, and diphtheria dropped significantly. Thanks to vaccinations, diseases like smallpox and rinderpest have been eradicated.[19] Polio is next in line, fingers crossed.

However, most other germs are not threatening our lives. Enough evidence shows us that killing as many germs as possible as frequently as possible just isn't working for human health. Today, the leading causes of death in humans are no longer infectious diseases, but chronic ones.[20] Cardiovascular diseases, cancer, COPD, dementia, and diabetes are responsible for more than half of the world's total deaths per year, with even higher rates in North America than elsewhere in the world.

The hygiene hypothesis, developed in 1989 by British epidemiology professor David Strachan, pointed out that exposure to infection was in fact beneficial to human health. In particular, exposure to microbes that have evolved alongside us for hundreds and thousands of years—in untreated water, in the dirt, in the animals we raise, and in the siblings we play with—benefits us.[21] Our bodies get used to these microbes in childhood, which helps us regulate our immune system.

This concept was further explored by specialists in allergies and immunology, and it gradually evolved into a broader hypothesis: declining microbial exposure is a major cause of the increasing incidence of atopy in recent years. Atopy, also known as "atopic or allergic march" as mentioned earlier, is a condition in which the body's immune system reacts to things it shouldn't. The condition is manifested in a progression (hence, a march) of allergic diseases. It first starts with eczema, progresses to hay fever and asthma, and then into food allergies.

Translated into nonresearch jargon: our kids are overcleaned, and they are not interacting with germs enough. As a result, their immune systems are malfunctioning.

The decreased microbial diversity and disrupted microbiome are not only linked to greater incidences of atopy, but also to other chronic inflammatory conditions, such as type 1 diabetes, multiple sclerosis, and inflammatory bowel disease.[22] When our body lacks a proper mix of symbiotic microorganisms, our immune system doesn't work properly. When this happens, substances that are not enemies to our body trigger immune responses that cause us pain and discomfort.

Humans know so little about 99.99% of the organisms on the planet—namely, the microorganisms. Each of us bears billions and trillions of microbes within us, and they are not free-riders, nor are they of no concern to us. They are our best friends and our deadliest enemies. Some of them digest our food and clean our guts while others cause illnesses and epidemics.[23]

Scientist and doctor of gastroenterology Dr. Giulia Enders explained in her TED Talk, "The Surprisingly Charming Science of Your Gut":

> We have 100 trillion bacteria doing all sorts of things in and on our body, and we need to understand bacteria differently. The research we have today is creating a new definition of what real cleanliness is. When you have too little microbes in your environment because you clean all the time, that's not a good thing because people get more allergies or autoimmune diseases. Hygiene is not about killing off bacteria right away. When we look at the facts, 95% of all bacteria on this planet don't harm us—they can't, they don't have the genes to do so. Many actually help us a lot, and scientists at the moment are looking into things like: Do some bacteria help us clean the gut? Do they help us digest? Do they make us put on weight or have a lean figure? Are others making us feel more courageous or even more resilient to stress? So there are more questions when it comes to cleanliness. We can't avoid the bad all the time. This is simply not possible because there's always something bad around. Our immune system needs the bad, too, so it knows what it's looking out for.

As babies and small children, our skin tries to grow and mature. This requires the right environment, one that is hygienic and natural, with friendly microorganisms and without pathogenic germs and chemicals. A hygienic and natural environment is the best way for our skin to strengthen its immune system so it knows how to respond as our world gets dirtier and more complicated. So, to help your children and their skin, use as few chemical products on their delicate skin as possible, and wash with just water daily. This will give them the best chance to develop a strong immune system with few or no allergies. That *is* good hygiene.

And for elders who feel dry and itchy or red and scaly? Is it just their bad health and old skin causing these conditions? Or is it the same *Skin Sobering* theory, requiring the same skin care practices? Frail elders and babies share one common bond: they depend upon you to take care of them. So, your knowledge and skin care practices don't just affect your own beauty and health.

When my dad was terminally ill and bedridden, my mom and I shampooed and washed him daily, lathering him lovingly with moisturizers that claimed to help sensitive skin. Though we had the best intentions, my Baba died itching. I wish I had known better.

I am not clean-obsessed, nor an opponent of germ theory. My dad was a pediatrician, and my mom was an obstetrician-gynecologist. Their practices saved many lives, so I believe in medicine, both Western and Eastern. I cannot tolerate disorganization in my office or home, but I can endure my floor not being mopped for weeks. I can wear the same apron for a month, and I'll work in my garden for a whole day and only wash my hands before I cook or eat.

I believe to maintain optimal health we need to build that health within our body, our cells, and in our immune system. We also need to be *hygienic* and get rid of harmful germs, using methods that don't further harm our bodies. For example, cleaning with water and pure soap on parts of our body that touch public surfaces is a wonderful way to accomplish this.

I am also aware of the increasing prevalence of highly resistant strains of "superbugs," and that it is due to the overuse and inappropriate use of antibiotics. This is eerily similar to the epidemic of skin diseases and beauty problems caused by cleaning and caring products. It is time to realize our beliefs about cleanliness were most likely influenced by, if not entirely born out of, marketing and promotions.

PROMOTE. PROMOTE. PROMOTE.

Location, location, location is the mantra for real estate sales. In the beauty industry, it is *promote, promote, promote.*

The beauty and skincare industry is one of the world's most profitable industrial sectors,[24] dominated by big corporations and filled out by innumerable small players. Just one company, P&G, has more than 100,000 employees. Many of these employees sincerely want to help consumers. They enter the industry with a strong aspiration to develop and sell products that improve people's lives and satisfy their needs. However, both corporations and locally owned mom-and-pop shops exist for another purpose: to make money. These companies create products to satisfy the needs of their shareholders first. The structure of the industry and the principles of economics get in the way of skin health.

The annual sales of this massive industry is somewhere between $250 and $400 billion, depending on where you draw the line between product sectors. By 2026, that number is expected to reach $756 billion.[25] Again, we're talking *annual* sales! Naturally, their promotional dollars are in the billions as well.

Here's a quick list of the major players, their 2021 revenue,[26] and their well-known brands:

L'Oréal
Revenue: $33.93 billion
Brands: Maybelline New York, Garnier, Lancôme, Vichy, Biotherm, Shu Uemura, Kiehl's, Dermablend, The Body Shop, Skinceuticals, La-Roche-Posay, Urban Decay

Unilever Group
Revenue: $25.38 billion

Brands: Dove, Sunsilk, Axe, Rexona, Lux, Pond's, Dermalogica, Degree, Pears

The Proctor & Gamble Co (after dropping around 100 brands by 2014)
Revenue: $19.41 billion
Brands: Olay, Head & Shoulders, Herbal Essences, Pantene, SK-II, Noxzema, Max Factor

Estee Lauder Co. Inc.
Revenue: $14.29 billion
Brands: Clinique, Prescriptives, Origins, M-A-C, Bobbi Brown, La Mer, Aveda, GoodSkin, Smashbox

If the above list of companies and brand names sound astounding, the huge varieties within the same brand will make your head spin. Variety sells. Let's choose Olay. Here are the different products bearing the Olay brand:

1. Olay Regenerist Retinol24 Night Moisturizer
2. Olay Eyes Retinol24 Night Eye Cream
3. Olay Regenerist Retinol24 Night Facial Serum
4. Olay Serums Pressed Serum Stick Refreshing
5. Olay Serums Pressed Serum Stick Cooling Hydration
6. Olay Total Effects Whip Face Moisturizer SPF 25 Fragrance-Free
7. Olay Regenerist Whip Face Moisturizer
8. Olay Eyes Brightening Eye Cream for Dark Circles
9. Olay Eyes Pro Retinol Eye Treatment for Wrinkles
10. Olay Eyes Ultimate Eye Cream for Wrinkles, Puffy Eyes and Dark Circles
11. Olay Eyes Eye Lifting Serum for Sagging Skin
12. Olay Sensitive Calming Facial Moisturizer SPF 15

13. Olay Sensitive Calming Liquid Cleanser with Hungarian Water Essence
14. Olay Sensitive Calming Cleansing Water, Fragrance-Free
15. Olay Sensitive Makeup Remover Wipes with Hungarian Water Essence
16. Olay Sensitive Calming Liquid Cleanser
17. Olay Glow Boost White Charcoal Clay Face Mask Stick
18. Olay Glow Boost Black Charcoal Clay Face Mask Stick
19. Olay ProX Microdermabrasion Plus Advanced Cleansing System

...

...

76. Olay Regenerist Micro-Sculpting Eye Swirl Eye Cream, Eye Treatment
77. Olay Total Effects Anti-Aging Eye Treatment
78. Olay Regenerist Instant Fix Wrinkle and Pore Vanisher

The above listed just 20 of almost 80 products Olay offers for skin care, for the face alone.

Again, this is *one* label from *one* brand under *one* company. Before P&G implemented its refocusing strategy to reduce its brands from 170 to 65, it was the world's largest single advertiser, spending a whopping $11.5 *billion* a year,[27] every year, on marketing, to convince people that they need P&G's products. In today's social media craze, with more influencers to influence consumers, these companies' marketing dollars are only increasing. Of course, its competitors did the same—their options were to either spend billions in promotion to compete or to die out.

These promotional and marketing strategies are not just a fine-tuned art. They have also incorporated well-tested *science* from psychology and behavioral economics. *Horizontal segmentation*, a niche market approach pioneered by American market research guru Howard Moskowitz, is a well-exercised strategy. With horizontal segmentation, companies alter the smell, color, flavor, package, function, or any minor aspect they can think of to cater to a slightly different niche of consumer preference. Fragrances and colors sell. By simply adding new scents to a product, brands can create the illusion of an entirely new product line. Varieties create new markets, varieties create more sales, and varieties create renewed hope. Why wouldn't you believe that you need all these hope-inducing products when they create so many more possibilities for you? The same trick is used for cars, fashion, food, and many other products we see, use, and think about every day.

The average North American woman puts 16 different products on her face in the morning.[28] Using a conservative calculation, this would be a cost of about $8 a day or up to $300,000 on skin care throughout her lifetime. All these products mean more ingredients, more fragrances, more botanicals, more preservatives, more surfactants, more potential for more reactions—invisible and visible—and, ultimately, more skin problems.

Consumers then buy more products, hoping to fix these skin problems.

When the products don't work, they're thrown out and replaced with new ones.

How many Olay products are a result of horizontal segmentation? I've lost count. These products have such similar names, I had to use Microsoft Word's number formatting tool to help me count. As of this book's publication, the answer is: 78 products from one brand, *and that's only the facial products*. There are 31 additional products if you include those meant for your body, for a total of 109 products. If all or any of these products truly worked, wouldn't our related beauty "problems" have gone away by now? *Source: Olay's own official website. There were actually 146 total products. My combing attempt didn't catch them all.*[29]

New products enter the market almost daily, and all of them claim to be game-changing. It's not uncommon for people to want to try the latest and greatest thing, especially if they think it will solve a problem. However, experienced physicians and surgeons have pleaded with their patients to not try any new technique, device, or procedure that has not been widely used for at least a year.[30] This shouldn't exclude products.

Of note: *never* buy a product or device that promises to reverse facial aging. Experienced medical practitioners have witnessed beauty-altering, "revolutionary" products come onto the market with a bang only to practically disappear a year later when real-world application proved them useless. *Big thunder little rain*—雷聲大雨點小 (lei sheng da yu dian xiao). Overpromise, underdeliver.

THE LEGAL VACUUM

So, who tells us if any product really works and how well it works? Not the Food and Drug Administration (FDA). The FDA only approves safety, but it is not responsible for conducting the safety tests. The beauty companies are. The beauty companies can also make many "magical" claims, which they are quite skilled at by presenting information that appears to support them. These are all allowed by the FDA.

Skin and beauty companies are not only allowed to make their life-changing claims, but they are in charge of testing and providing proof of those claims. The conflict of interest here is blatantly clear. Further, these companies have an obligation to their shareholders to first recover the FDA approval costs, then to turn a major profit. To make this happen, they market the hell out of their products in any way they can. Their goal is to convince us we need their products, and they'll say and do almost anything to make us feel that way. Their company's financial bottom line is and always will be their primary concern. This attitude is resulting in global, widespread skin issues.

And no one is stopping them.

SKINCARE PRODUCTS AND DRUGS

I really don't want to talk about skincare products and medicinal drugs together, as it infers that our beauty problem is a disease. It also reinforces the concept that there's something wrong with our skin, which perpetuates this obsession of having to fix it with something. But I do want to make an important point: the products we use to treat our skin beauty issues should be treated like drugs! There are a few skincare products that actually can improve some beauty conditions, but they must be used according to a well-managed regimen and only for a limited time, just like medicine, because of their risks and side effects.

In 1938, President Franklin Roosevelt signed the Food, Drug, and Cosmetic Act into law, granting the US FDA the power to regulate food, drugs, and cosmetics. While the new law prohibited *false claims* for drugs, a separate law was passed giving the Federal Trade Commission (FTC) jurisdiction over advertising. This transpired shortly after an advertised "miracle elixir" (antifreeze) killed several people, many of whom were children. At the same time, a dozen users of a mascara called "Lash Lure" went blind from exposure to the toxic chemical paraphenylenediamine (PPD), otherwise commonly found in permanent hair dye.

Today, the FDA officially defines a cosmetic as "A product (excluding pure soap) intended to be applied to the human body for cleansing, beautifying, promoting attractiveness, or altering the appearance." And a drug is defined as "A substance (other than food) intended to affect the structure or any function of the body."[31] These definitions are almost word-for-word the same as they were when the law was passed in 1938, yet in the last 80 years, cosmetic ingredients, chemistry, and the industry have changed greatly. Using an outdated definition to govern an ever-changing industry is cause for significant concern.

Here is an example of how cosmetic *chemistry* has changed: In the 1980s, doctors Eugene J. Van Scott and Ruey J. Yu patented alpha hydroxy acid (AHA),[32] an ingredient found in sour milk (lactic acid) that was allegedly used by Cleopatra. Van Scott and Yu showed that AHA could "thin very thick skin by exfoliation, plump up skin by increasing the water-binding materials naturally found in skin, and help minimize lines and wrinkles by stimulating the production of collagen, giving the skin a stronger base." All of these claims are wonderful *and* demonstrate an *"altering of [the skin's] structure and function"*—which, by the FDA's own definition, should mean that AHA is classified as a drug. Yet, it is not! AHAs and many other active ingredients remain a loosely regulated, cosmetic product and do not have to adhere to drug regulations. AHAs have contributed over a billion dollars annually to anti-aging skincare sales.

Conversely, petroleum jelly—100% petrolatum (commonly known as Vaseline)—was shown in the 1970s to change severe dry and cracked skin to a soft and supple texture. Afterward, petrolatum was included in the definition of "altering skin structure and functions" and was classified as a drug. If you buy a jar of Vaseline today, you will see that it actually has a drug fact label and is marketed as an over-the-counter (OTC) drug.

Vaseline is the most inert, least irritating substance you can put on your skin. It sits on top of your skin, creating a barrier to help prevent moisture loss without getting into your pores so sweat can still secrete. Vaseline is so purified that it's the only OTC substance used on burned skin to preserve moisture.

Inert petrolatum is a drug, but *active* AHAs don't have to follow drug regulations? This makes no sense.

M. Varinia Michalun and Joseph C. Dinardo (2015) summarized this better than anyone else in their book *Skin Care and Cosmetic Ingredients Dictionary*:

> Both AHAs and Petrolatum change the "structure and function" of skin. Both significantly impact the skin...Yet AHAs are sold as

cosmetics (~$150/10 fl. Oz) and 100% Petrolatum (~$3/10 fl. Oz) is sold as an OTC drug. What then permits the 1938 FDA law to classify them differently?...it is what the manufacturer *claims or says* about the product and its activity on the skin. Regardless whether the ingredients actually impact the skin's structure [or] function...regulations only apply if the product or ingredient(s) are discussed in ways that can be interpreted as a drug or pharmaceutical claim. AHA-based products are sold as skin moisturizers, and their packaging and advertising will generally read: "apply this luxuriously rich moisturizing cream day and night for younger more radiant *looking* skin." This is a cosmetic claim because it refers to "altering the appearance" of the skin—that is, skin looks more youthful and radiant. It is not claiming to *make* the skin more youthful and radiant. In the case of Petrolatum, [they] usually state "for the temporary relief of chapped skin or lips." This is a drug claim because it refers to "altering the structure" of your skin.

    The 1938 FDA law has not kept up with science. Our understanding about what happens in skin when an ingredient or product is applied to it has become extremely advanced. These capacities did not exist when the FDA developed its law. Today, one can say that almost all ingredients impact the "structure or function" of the skin one way or another. This being the case, it would appear that the only way the FDA can enforce the 1938 Food, Drug, and Cosmetic Act is by either establishing "logical standards" which would require receiving a significant increase in resources (funding, equipment, and personnel); or by continuing to let the cosmetic industry regulate itself. The cost to redefine this almost 200-billion-dollar global industry is more than most governments are willing to do. This is especially the case since the cosmetic industry has caused very minimal problems worldwide.[33]

These authors made excellent points, but "minimal problems"? Only if we don't consider eczema, dermatitis, psoriasis, sensitivity, dryness, oiliness, and acne, *problems*; or if we don't think spending $300,000 in a lifetime based on false hopes and misleading advertisements is problematic; or if we decide we don't care that skin problems are the number one reason Americans visit their doctors.[34]

To complicate matters, as mentioned earlier, the FDA also put the responsibility of proving product safety on the cosmetic manufacturers. If the manufacturer does not test the product and demonstrate that it is safe, they can still *market* and *sell* the product. They simply have to add a small warning label to the product that states, "The safety of this product has not been determined." Do most people read the fine print?

Look closely at that warning. Notice it is about product *safety*, not product *efficacy*, let alone product *effectiveness*. And safety is usually measured in a specific timeframe. So if something doesn't cause harm in the short run, even if it does so down the road, it could still be labeled as safe. Efficacy is showing a beneficial change under ideal and controlled circumstances, and effectiveness refers to a product's performance under real-world conditions. Skincare and cosmetic products should prove their *effectiveness* when they make any beneficial claims—or at least show efficacy—but the FDA doesn't require any of this from companies. The responsibility of providing product information is completely on the same manufacturers who make almost all their decisions based on maximizing profit.

Today, many products contain biologically active ingredients. They are cleverly named "cosmeceuticals," a combination of "cosmetics" and "pharmaceuticals" that serves the exact purpose of *implying* the product is more than just a cosmetic—it is *pharmaceutical* grade, you know! In a way, they are right, actually. These products are drugs to your skin. They can interact with the body's biochemical mechanisms and alter your skin. They go far beyond the 1938 FDA definition, but they don't have to adhere to modern regulations governing "real" drugs.

This slippery marketing tactic is really the best of both worlds for the cosmetic industry: follow the loose, self-regulated cosmetic act, but claim the pharmaceutical effects of the drug act to minimize investment and maximize sales. This is a win-win situation for them, but not for consumers.

What does all this mean for you?

Imagine if a whole class of drugs was able to get away with calling themselves food (or lotion), for example, and had billions of marketing dollars to influence you to absorb as much of it as possible as frequently as possible, double dose it, multilayer it, and never go without it. And imagine if cigarette advertisers were still allowed to influence people by only highlighting the positive effects of tobacco, like it can lift your spirits, make you feel cool, curb your appetite so you can lose weight, and more, all without including any warning statements. People would feel quite encouraged to pick up smoking, as they were in the past when this advertising was allowed in that industry. Worse, those positive claims aren't exactly untrue—people actually do experience those sensations—but while they are real, they are fleeting, impermanent, and damaging.

When it comes to tobacco and drugs, the law has changed to force these companies to be more honest. As a result, these companies are no longer legally allowed to withhold information about harm and long-term damage. Unfortunately, for the beauty industry, the law is loosey-goosey, and skincare companies are still marketing however they want. They are happy to advertise all their *apparent* benefits (whether or not the supposed benefits are even there after the product is off), and they aren't obligated to mention anything about inherent harm.

Drugs are not all bad, but they are bad for you if you treat them as nutrients, indulge, or neglect to follow the proper usage guidelines.

Most cosmetic ingredients will never be banned. They are not toxic, per se. Even tobacco is not banned. So, how could we justify banning minor offenders present in modern-day cosmetics? The best we can do is to try to understand that skincare products are simply *not beneficial to us*.

Remember, this industry is powerful, and consumers love innovation. The beauty and skincare industries have research teams and marketing departments ready to replace any questionable ingredients and repackage the same products as new and improved. These companies also have the best and most resourceful legal teams and lobbyists in their corner, prepared to deflect any consumer complaints. After all, a great way to quiet a disgruntled consumer is to refund their money and gift them a sample of a brand-new goodie. Surely this one will transform your skin, right? How brilliant.

SKINCARE PRODUCTS SHOULD AT LEAST BE TREATED AS MAKEUP

I will not be able to change FDA regulations to have them classify skincare products as drugs. Elle Woods (in *Legally Blonde*) couldn't achieve that either, despite her legal and beauty sassiness. But I think the following is possible: skincare products should at least be treated like makeup products!

Makeup is quite amazing. It makes you look illuminated, smooth, and a different color. Makeup is essentially paint, and its application can be considered an art. Interestingly, we tend to have a much healthier relationship with makeup than with skincare products. We know how makeup can help our face and how it can harm it. Therefore, we typically maintain a healthy distance with makeup and make sure we take it off before bed. We don't leave it on to let the "beauty nutrients" penetrate. So, although makeup causes the same harm as skincare products, it is in some ways less harmful because we use it less and clean it off sooner.

Skincare products, like cleansers and lotions, are much more harmful than makeup because we have been led to believe they are capable of providing nutrients to the skin. We use them to remove makeup, double cleanse, then moisturize, nourish, protect, and then we leave them on the skin to permeate their goodness. But in reality, we are allowing the colorless (or flesh-colored) substances to soak into our skin all day and all night.

That's insane. And that's the reason why skincare products are much worse than makeup—the 24/7 long wear and constant attack!

2

EVIDENCE

WHAT SCIENTISTS AND DOCTORS (WHO DON'T SELL PRODUCTS) SAY ABOUT OUR SKIN

STRUCTURE AND FUNCTION OF THE SKIN
*An Excretory (Waste-Elimination) Organ • The Skin You See •
Dead Cells Fall Willingly, New Cells Come Naturally • The Billion-Dollar Creation—NMF •
Our Skin Army • The Lush Skin Geography*

A SUMMARY AND SOME UTTER BS
Can the Skin Absorb Nutrients? • Moisturization. Exfoliation. Sensitivity.

FROM THE ANTI-AGING DOCTOR

In 1999, I started a skin health clinic specializing in facial skin analysis using microscopic examination. I have always believed that skin examinations are as important as physical or mental examinations and should not be neglected. My method caught media attention, and many patients flocked to my practice to receive this service. Thanks to them,

Figure A: **Microscopic Examination Data 1999**

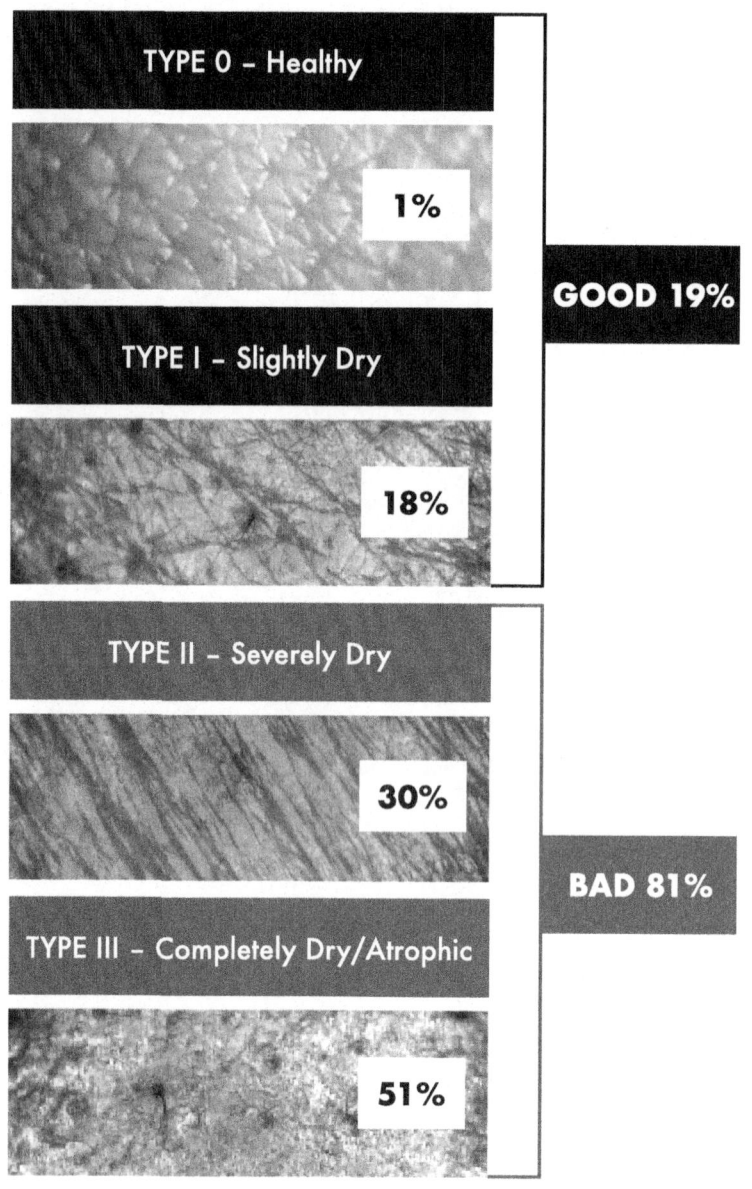

TYPE 0 – Healthy

1%

TYPE I – Slightly Dry

18%

GOOD 19%

TYPE II – Severely Dry

30%

TYPE III – Completely Dry/Atrophic

51%

BAD 81%

Note: Results based on 100 consecutive cases

I very quickly collected large numbers of data. Analyzing this data produced some unexpected findings.

The first set of data was collected from 207 women in 1999.[35] The examination results showed that 81% (168) of the women had severe dry or dehydrated skin (Type II & III, in Figure A), and 51% (105) had the worst, completely dry, atrophic problems (Type III). Only 18% (37) had somewhat normal, slightly dry skin (Type I), and a mere 1% (2) had healthy, problem-free skin (Type 0).

As seen under a microscope, the healthy Type 0 condition has a grainy texture made up of numerous tiny mounds and grooves in an orderly network. Doctors refer to this as the "dermatoglyphics" 肌理 or "grains of the skin" (Figure B). These healthy grains appear to the naked eye as supple, hydrated, and smooth skin. If the dermatoglyphics disappear, a long list of aesthetic and health issues can arise.

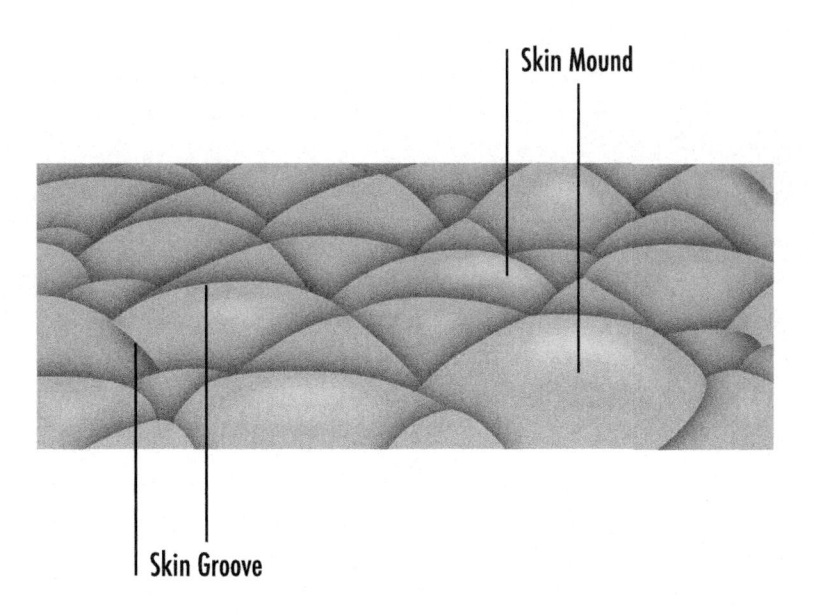

Figure B: **Dermatoglyphics**

Skin Mound

Skin Groove

How bad was the most severe Type III skin of the 105 people? Their skin had completely lost the grains otherwise found in healthy skin. The mounds and grooves had flattened, and the grains were no longer visible. Their skin was shriveling and atrophying because there was very little cell division and regeneration. You could not *see* the problems with the naked eye, especially when products were masking the condition. Even so, the person could *feel* it—dry and pulled (especially when the moisturizers were washed off)—and the microscope could pick it up. The condition almost mimicked a collagen disease or the thin membrane of a blister. This is very sick skin, and it was shocking to find it was present in such a large proportion of my patients. I could hardly believe this, and I thought there must be something wrong with my examination.

The people who participated in these examinations did not neglect their skin. They cared enough to pay ¥35,000 ($300 USD) to spend an hour and get an expert analysis. If anything, they were more concerned about their skin than the average person, but why then did almost all of them have problematic skin? And among these people, more than half had such severe damage that their skin cells were no longer regenerating! When I examined their skin and skin care behavior further, I discovered that those who were keen on skincare products and beauty routines had worse skin. Their skin was drier, oilier, rougher, duller, and/or dehydrated. Basically, they were experiencing an exacerbation of whatever *inherent* issues they already had.

Clinical data was continuously collected on patients seeking skin analysis. In 2016, a study was published comparing the skin of 100 patients before *Skin Sobering* and 30 days after[36] (Figure C1 and C2). Before *Skin Sobering*, only two patients had Type 0 skin, and six had Type I skin. That is, 8% of people had "Good" normal skin (Type 0 and I). The number of patients with Type II skin was 28 and Type III was 64. That means 92% of them had "Bad" skin (Type II and III). After 30 days of *Skin Sobering*, those with "Bad" skin dropped from 92 to 57 people, a

Figure C1: **Microscoping Examination Data 2016**
(Before Skin Sobering)

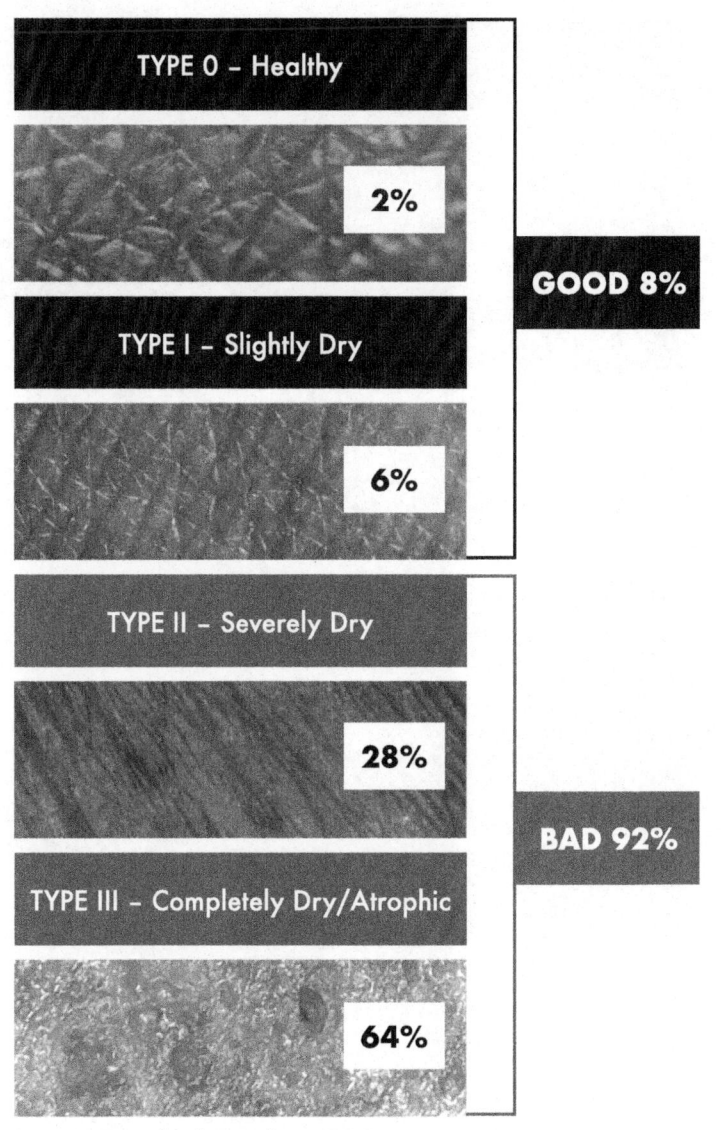

TYPE 0 – Healthy	
2%	GOOD 8%
TYPE I – Slightly Dry	
6%	
TYPE II – Severely Dry	
28%	BAD 92%
TYPE III – Completely Dry/Atrophic	
64%	

Note: Results based on 100 consecutive cases

EVIDENCE • 27

Figure C2: **Microscoping Examination Data 2016**
(After Skin Sobering)

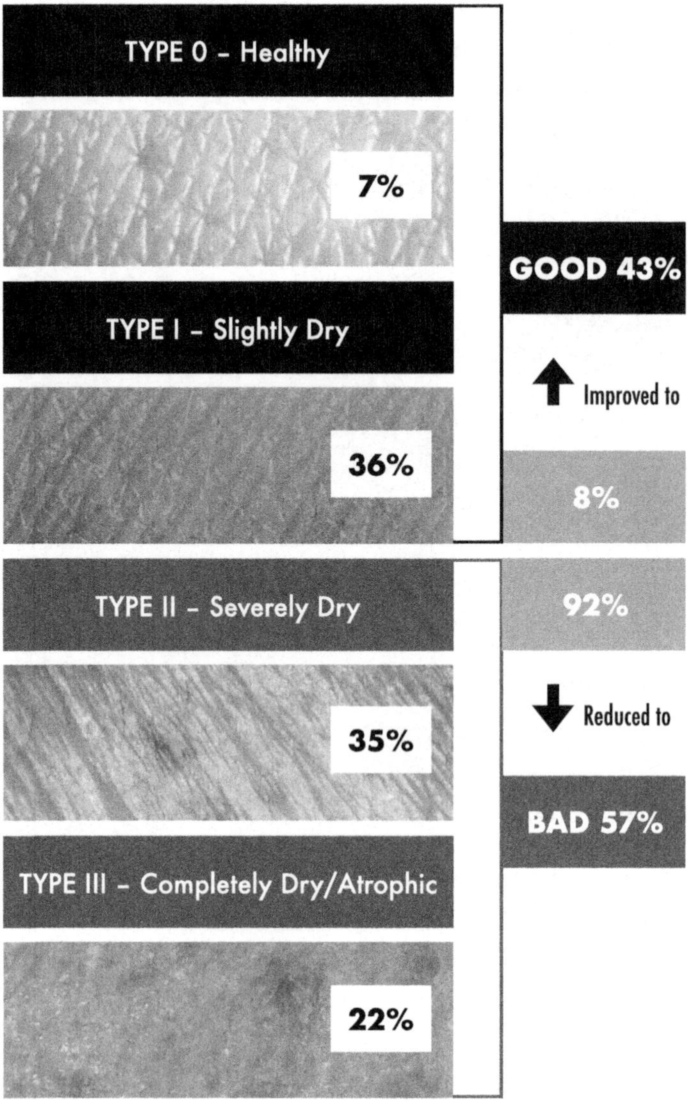

Type	%
TYPE 0 – Healthy	7%
TYPE I – Slightly Dry	36%
TYPE II – Severely Dry	35%
TYPE III – Completely Dry/Atrophic	22%

GOOD 43% ⬆ Improved to 8%

92% ⬇ Reduced to **BAD 57%**

Note: *Results based on 100 consecutive cases*

61% reduction. Conversely, those with "Good" skin increased from 8 to 43 people, a 437% improvement.

This reported data and the thousands more that was collected demonstrated a complete contradiction of what we have been told, what has been marketed to us, and what we cosmetic doctors have been doing to patients. I presented these findings to the Japanese Society of Aesthetic Dermatology, the International Society of Aesthetic Plastic Surgery, and many other scientific conferences.[37,38,39,40,41,42] I wanted the world to know this!

STRUCTURE AND FUNCTION OF THE SKIN

AN EXCRETORY (WASTE-ELIMINATION) ORGAN

Let's take a look at the skin in a simple and functional way. This will be the most scientifically complex portion of the book, but please do not skip past it. Once you have an understanding of how your skin works, you will clearly understand how and why skincare products are damaging it.

The skin is our body's largest organ, and it is an excretory one. If we could spread out the skin of an adult, it would cover about 2 square meters. Its total weight is about 3 to 4 kilograms, so it is also the body's heaviest organ.

Excretion is the process of removing waste and excess water from the body, to maintain internal chemical homeostasis and prevent toxin accumulation. The well-known organs and parts in our body that also carry out this vital role are the kidneys, liver, lungs, large intestine, salivary glands, urethra, and anus. What few people know is that the skin also fulfills this excretory role.

All living organisms must eliminate the wastes that result from metabolism, and they expel the broken-down components in the form of solids, liquids, or gas. Otherwise, they will die. We know that feces and urine are waste, but so are breath, gas, saliva, nasal fluid, tears, vaginal discharge, and sweat. Not all the body's biological by-products are bad or gross. Many of them have important protective and beneficial functions. We are quite aware of the benefits of nasal fluid, saliva, and tears, but lesser known by-products like discharge, sweat, and sebum are also beneficial.

Humans and other mammals are the only organisms that can excrete sweat through the pores of the skin to get rid of oil, urea, salt, sugar, and ammonia. This is one group of "waste" that needs to leave our body, but it also has important protective functions for our skin. If excretion doesn't happen in an unobstructed manner, thoroughly and smoothly, we don't feel good, and we don't look well. A constipated person, or a person holding her pee or breath, looks visibly uncomfortable. We know this, so we don't ever intentionally obstruct these organs, nor their excretory holes. We don't dare to block the anus, urethra, or nose—the large, singular excretory hole—but what about the millions of tiny, easily clogged openings on our skin—our pores? These are *also* excretory openings! Why do so many people obstruct them daily and continuously? Do they even know that's what they are doing?

Layers of the Skin

The skin has a thin layer on the surface called the epidermis and a thick layer in the middle called the dermis (Figure D). Underneath them are the supporting hypodermis and muscles. The epidermis is only about 0.4–0.7 millimeters thick. In other words, it has roughly the same thickness as a piece of clear plastic food wrap. The epidermis is further divided into several sublayers. Even though these are viable cells and metabolically active, the epidermal layer has no blood vessels to give its cells nutrients, nor lymph vessels to process waste.[43] Yet, these cells continue to metabolize and function. It is quite remarkable.

The dermis is about 10 to 40 times thicker than the epidermis. It is primarily composed of collagen and elastin fibers and the fibroblast cells that produce these fibers. The dermis also gives the skin its

Figure D: **Layers of the Skin**

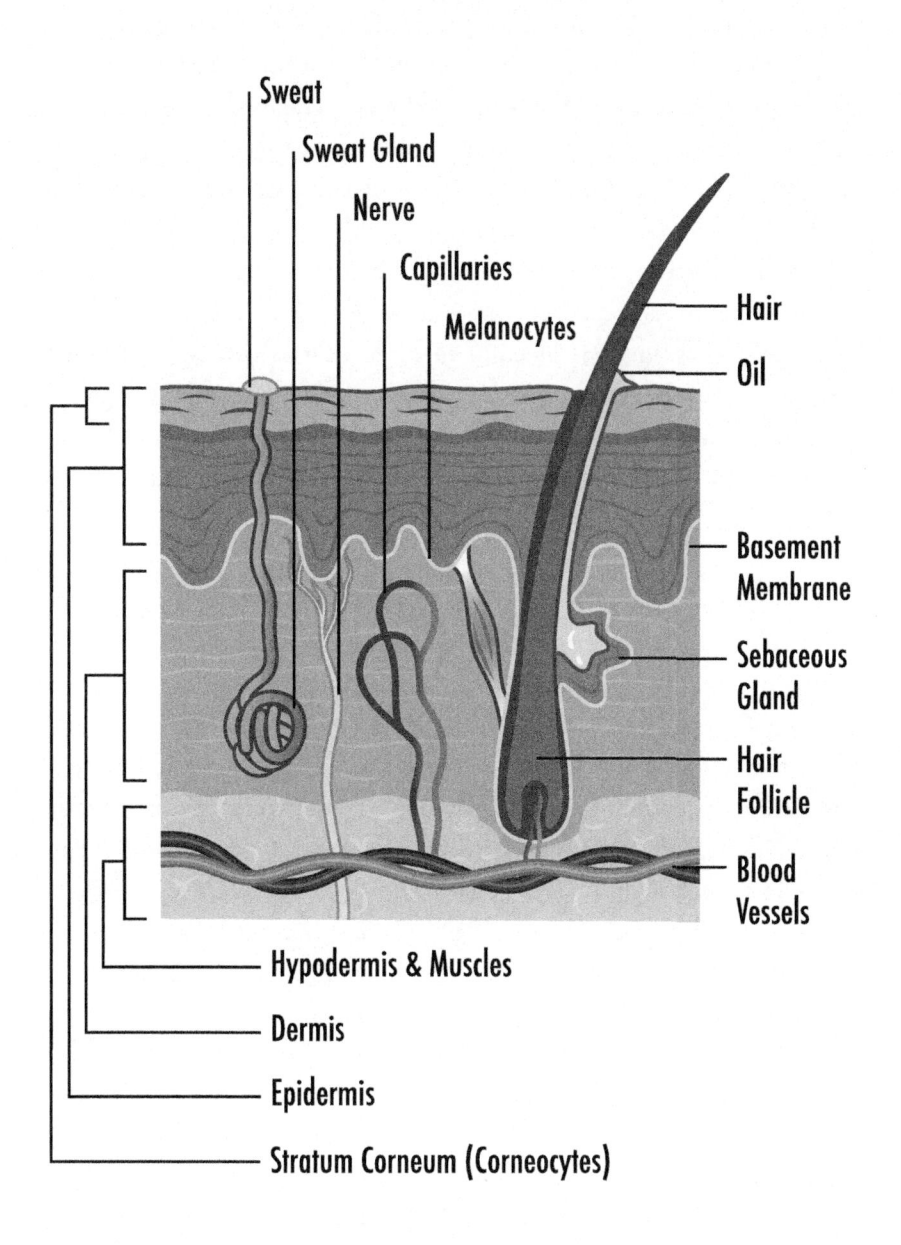

- Sweat
- Sweat Gland
- Nerve
- Capillaries
- Melanocytes
- Hair
- Oil
- Basement Membrane
- Sebaceous Gland
- Hair Follicle
- Blood Vessels
- Hypodermis & Muscles
- Dermis
- Epidermis
- Stratum Corneum (Corneocytes)

structural framework, strength, elasticity, and suppleness. If you don't already know, leather that is used to make shoes and clothes is the dermis of animals. You can see how resilient the dermis is. The dermis also houses a crisscrossing network of blood vessels, lymphatic vessels, nerve fibers, oil and sweat glands, and hair follicles, where the supply of nutrients and removal of wastes happen. This network of content is very pigmented—blue, gray, red, dark. Our fingerprints are also determined by the dermis, despite the prints being on the outer layer.

As there are no blood vessels or nerve cells in the epidermis, if we scrape it, the skin won't bleed or feel pain. There will be no scarring either, and healing is very fast. However, if the dermis is damaged, a complex healing process will take place and scarring can happen.

We won't discuss the hypodermis and muscle layers in the scope of this book.

THE SKIN YOU SEE

One important sublayer of the epidermis is the stratum corneum, also called the "horny layer" because its cells are tough like an animal's horn (Figure E). The stratum corneum is the outermost layer of the skin, and it's what we see as our skin. This means that the healthier your stratum corneum, the prettier your skin appears. The stratum corneum is made up of "dead cells" called the corneocytes. It's been thought for a long time in dermatology that the corneocytes are dead, with no biological activity or function.[44] However, the current understanding is that the stratum corneum is a live tissue, and its corneocytes perform crucial protective and adaptive physiological functions.

The corneocytes are in the shape of a pentagon or hexagon, flat, and firmly cemented together in 15 to 20 layers to make the stratum corneum. The total thickness of the corneocytes' top layers is only 0.02 millimeters, so each individual layer is therefore incredibly thin and easily damaged. The corneocyte is the matured form of its precursor, the keratinocyte.

Figure E: **Sublayers of the Epidermis**

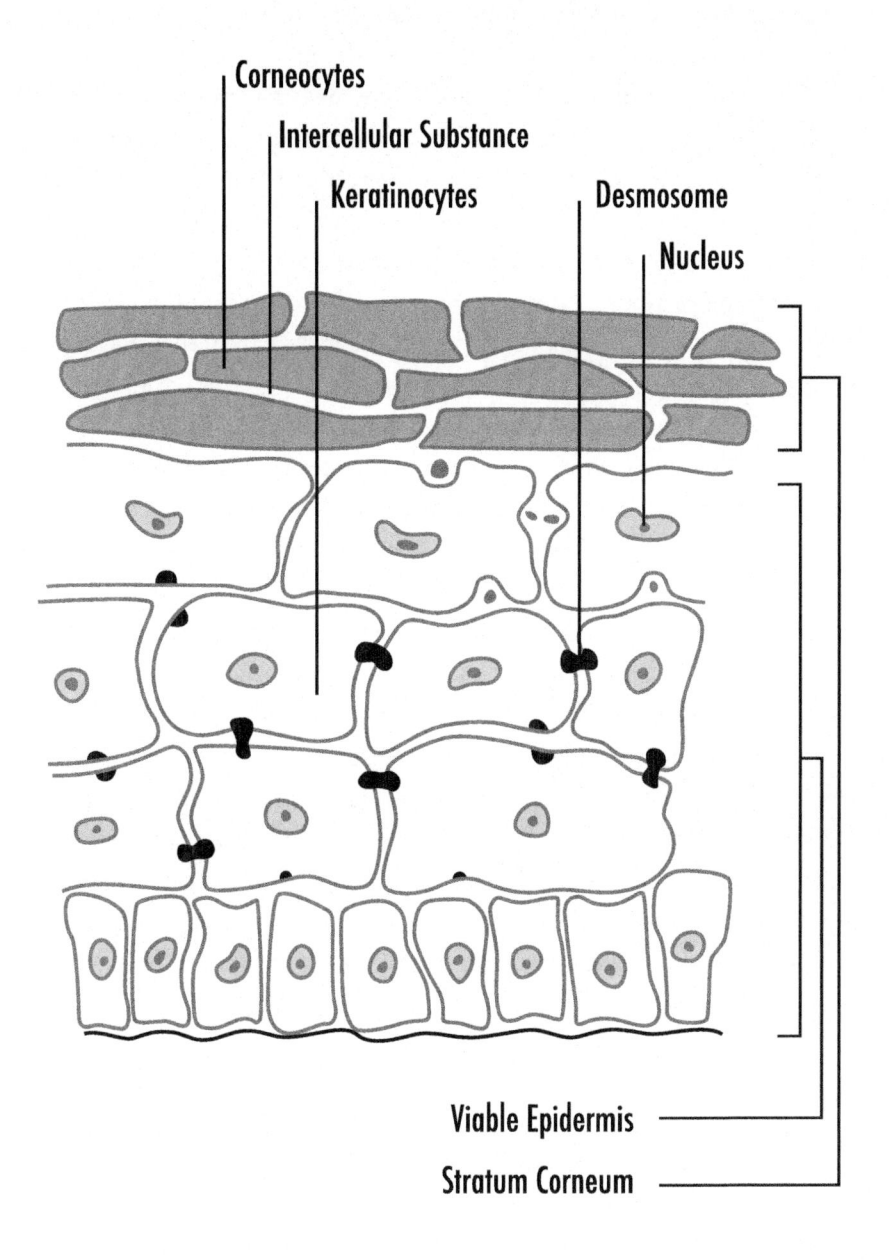

Corneocytes
Intercellular Substance
Keratinocytes
Desmosome
Nucleus

Viable Epidermis
Stratum Corneum

EVIDENCE · 33

When the keratinocyte "grows up" and loses its cellular contents (nucleus, water, amino acids), it becomes a corneocyte. The lost cellular contents fill the spaces between the corneocyte cells in the form of a matrix, which is made up of these water-soluble contents, and more—ceramides, cholesterol, and fatty acids. This water and lipid matrix form the intercellular substance (also known as the intercellular lamellar lipids). This substance binds the corneocytes together, making the stratum corneum a great barrier. Dermatology books often use the analogy of "bricks and mortar" to describe the stratum corneum—the corneocyte cells are the bricks, and the intercellular substance is the mortar. Together they form a tough, impermeable wall. This layer also carries out other important physiological functions including managing microbial growth, regulating hydration, controlling exfoliation, and initiating inflammation.[45]

When you examine the composition of the intercellular substance "mortar" using a microscope, you will find that it has a dual "lipid-water-lipid-water" configuration. The two opposing properties of lipid and water interlace with each other to achieve further hydration for the skin. Both the "bricks and mortar" structure and the lipid-water configuration of the mortar make the stratum corneum a dual structural wall and an outstanding moisture barrier. It can effectively prevent dehydration by stopping water from evaporating through the skin (transepidermal water loss—TEWL).[46] It can also inhibit foreign substances from penetrating the skin. The stratum corneum is the first line of defense for not only our skin but also our entire body—nothing foreign can come in, and precious moisture won't seep out.

DEAD CELLS FALL WILLINGLY, NEW CELLS COME NATURALLY

So, where does the corneocyte that makes up the stratum corneum come from? And how does the life cycle of skin cell turnover play out to make our skin beautiful?

Figure F: **Skin Cell Turnover of the Epidermis**

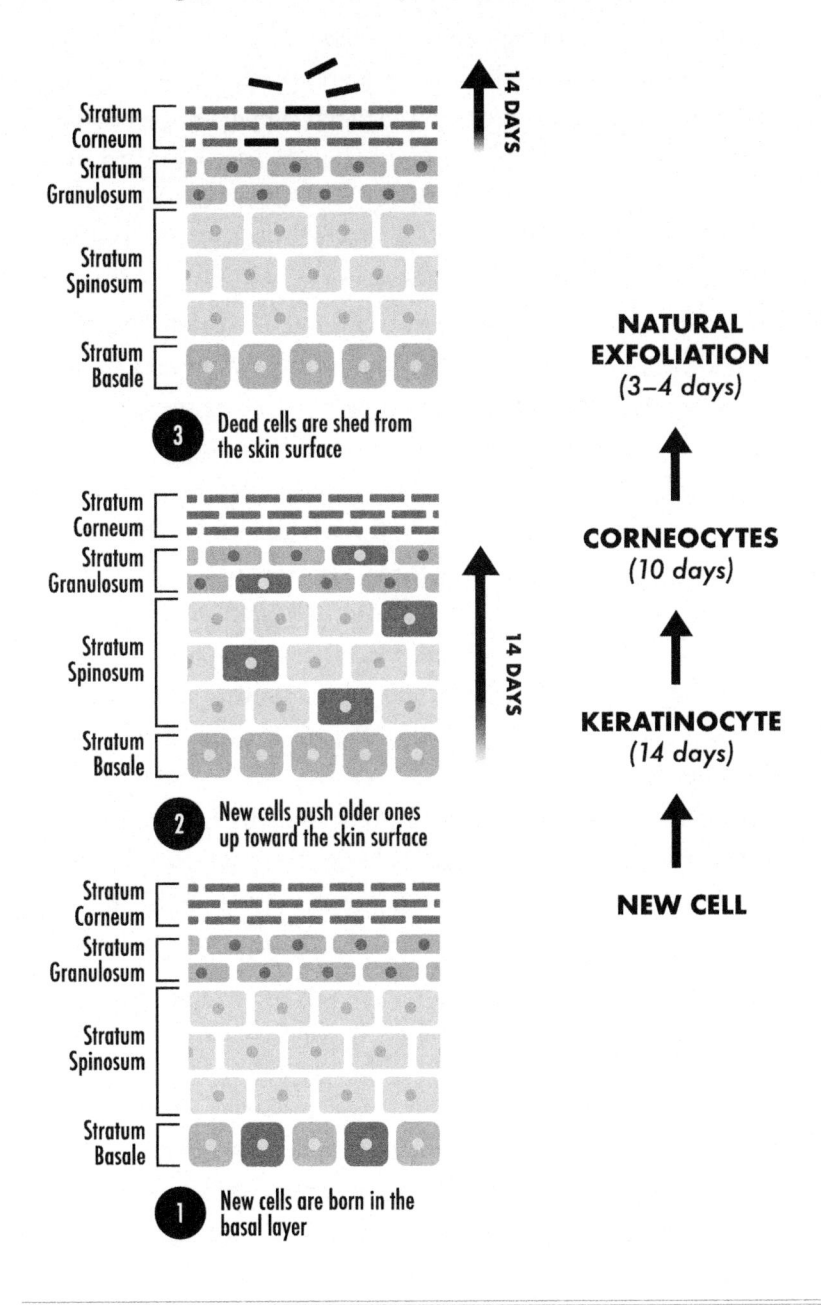

EVIDENCE • 35

Let's look at more layers of the epidermis (Figure F). The outermost layer is the stratum corneum, as we illustrated in Figure D. The base layer is the stratum basale (also called the stratum germinativum or the basal layer), which is the closest to the blood supply lying underneath the epidermis.[47] The cells of the germinativum continually divide (think germinate) through mitosis. In other words, the mother cell splits into two. The mother cell remains in the basale layer, and the newly divided cell is pushed upward toward the stratum corneum.[48,49] It takes about 14 days for the new cells to migrate from the basale layer to the bottom of the corneum layer. When the cells move upward, keratinocytes are formed first. Then they flatten, lose their water and cellular contents, and "die" to become corneocytes.

The "dead" corneocytes take about another 10 days to squeeze from the bottom of the stratum corneum to the surface. Once they've reached the surface, the neatly stacked corneocytes "bricks" that are held together by the "mortar" are exposed to the air for about three or four more days. During that time, they perform the crucial functions of preventing the skin from dehydration and protecting it against external invaders. Then, their mighty job is done. They are tired, and they slough off *on their own!*

This natural, continuous, turning-over mechanism is the infamous exfoliation of dead skin. Once the dead skin flakes and sloughs off, the cells underneath will migrate up and continue the same protective battle as their previous sisters-in-arms. This is the cycle of cell turnover and skin renewal, and it takes a total of about 28 days: 14 days for the divided cell to migrate to the base of the corneum layer; 10 days to move from the base to the top of the corneum; then 3 or 4 days to guard the surface before falling off. As we get older, our metabolism slows, and the migration can take longer than 28 days. Even though our metabolism will slow, it is critical that this turnover is not interfered with or disrupted in any way so our skin can renew optimally.

Critical Metabolic Signaling

The moment the top layer of dead skin is naturally falling off, an important and critical signal is sent back down to the stratum basale.[50] This signal tells it to make more new cells, and the signaling happens *only* when dead skin cells *naturally* slough off of their own volition. If they are not allowed to fall off when they are ready to, like if products have got them stuck together or *if you manually exfoliate them off*, the signal will not be sent and *no new cells will be made*!

This is the nature of our metabolism. Our skin can stay smooth because of its innate ability to control and manage the needs of many layers of the skin. We rely on this undisrupted metabolism for old cells to fall, new cells to divide, and for healthy, youthful skin to remain.

How do the dead corneocytes become fallen heroes, slough off stoically on their own, and send down the signal for new soldiers?

When the stratum corneum of normal skin makes direct contact with air, the corneocytes' edges will curl up, so more air can get underneath in order to lift and remove the tired cell. In about three days, this dead skin cell will naturally peel and fall off. It is at this exact moment that a signal is generated to the stratum basale layer to produce new cells. These new cells push themselves upward orderly and sequentially to replace the lost cells. This continuous falling off is what keeps the stratum corneum thin and smooth instead of becoming thick. The consistent production of new cells is what makes the epidermis plump and full.

Two desirable states of opposing anatomy, thin/smooth and plump/full, in the right layers result in evenness, suppleness, and the radiance that we see in healthy skin.

However, as soon as we use products (masks, serums, lotions, or creams), the skin surface becomes sticky. The edges of old corneocyte cells cannot get sufficient air exposure to curl up, making it difficult for these dead cells to lift and fall off. This means much less natural exfoliation is happening and far fewer metabolic signals are being sent down to generate new cells.

Can you picture what is going on with skin that is continuously covered in products? The stratum corneum cannot slough off naturally, exfoliation cannot happen, and cell regeneration is halted. What you see is a thick, rough, and dull stratum corneum and a thin, stiff, and weak epidermis. These are signs of atrophying skin. It's not nice on the eyes, and it's not good for your health.

Effective skin metabolism and renewal is vital and keeps skin healthy and beautiful. The skin needs to be in an airy, clear, and fresh state for this natural metabolic cycle of exfoliation and cell division to occur. Product-covered skin may temporarily appear to be smooth, but the product simultaneously impedes all the skin's natural functions. This impediment ultimately leads to many skin problems.

If you ever notice the skin of a young child (who hopefully hasn't started using many products yet), his or her skin does not feel sticky. It is clear, fresh, and dry to the touch. Yes, healthy skin should be dry—not the lacking-water or no-oil sort of dry, but clear, clean, and not sticky. When it comes to skin, it's hard to use the English word *dry* without bringing up negative connotations. We have a couple of better terms in Chinese, like 乾爽 / 清爽 (gan shuang/qing shuang)—meaning *dry fresh. Sober skin!* This is the best state for your skin to be in, as it will allow dead cells to exfoliate and slough off naturally. This allows your body to continuously create new cells.

Remember, good skin should not be sticky and moist. It should be clear and fresh. Don't add moisture or stickiness onto your skin! *Skin naturally desires sobriety.*

THE BILLION-DOLLAR CREATION—NMF

How our skin operates is nothing short of a miracle. Once you understand the wonders of your skin, you will realize why *not* using any products is the best way to keep this miracle going.

We already know that the skin is a *physical* barrier between the world and our internal organs and muscles. How is it also an amazing *moisture* barrier and a moisture *retainer*? These two properties not only come from the "bricks and mortar" formation, but also another magical substance: a biochemical material produced within the formation. This is called the natural moisturizing factor (NMF). (Figure G)

As you may recall, the brick-like corneocytes are keratinocytes with their water, nucleus, and cellular contents dissolved—think soybeans changing into miso beans. These dissolved contents, which are primarily amino acids, become the *water*-soluble moisturizing factor. In a parallel fashion, the mortar-like intercellular substance, which contains mostly fatty acids, turns into the *lipid*-soluble moisturizing factor. These two moisturizing factors then go through a maturing process during their upward migration to the surface of the stratum corneum and gain further moisturizing strength by combining and becoming the even mightier NMF. NMF also has an amazing ability to attract atmospheric water to further hydrate the skin.[51]

NMF's barrier function and moisturizing abilities are incredibly powerful, reaching the extremes of antidrought and antifreezing. Do you wonder why, when relative humidity in the air drops to below 10%, water underneath the skin does not vanish? Or why, when the temperature outside drops below 0 degrees Celsius, the skin does not freeze? It is because of NMF's phenomenal protective ability. Our skin will not dry up like a mummy's when we walk the Strip in Las Vegas, nor will it freeze like an icicle when we ski the Bushwacker in Telluride. Nature has given us a perfect blend of ingredients to protect our skin and our body, but we are trying to replace (and damage) this gift with chemicals!

Skincare companies know how powerful NMF is. They just choose not to talk about it or tell you about it. Instead, they spend millions in R&D and manufacturing trying to mimic NMF. No matter how much

Figure G: **Natural Moisturizing Factor (NMF)**

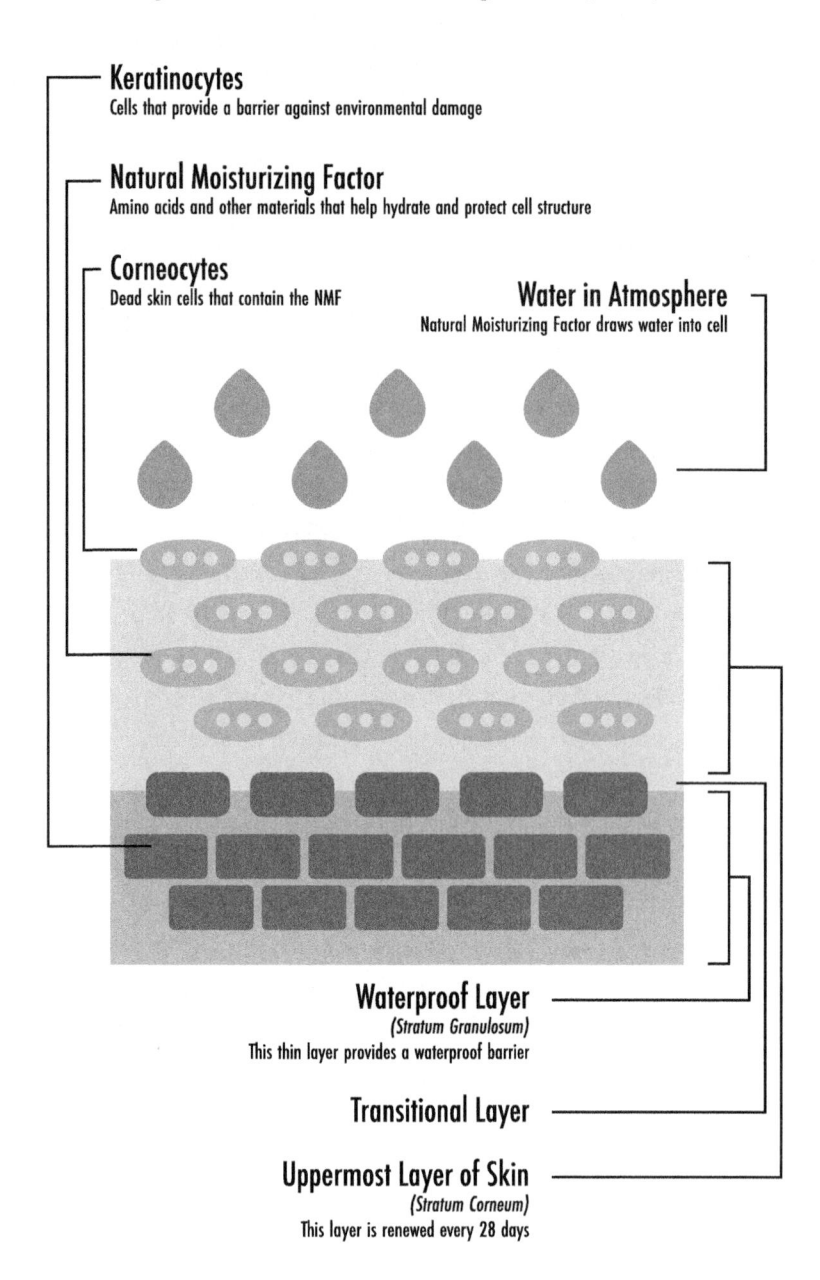

Keratinocytes
Cells that provide a barrier against environmental damage

Natural Moisturizing Factor
Amino acids and other materials that help hydrate and protect cell structure

Corneocytes
Dead skin cells that contain the NMF

Water in Atmosphere
Natural Moisturizing Factor draws water into cell

Waterproof Layer
(Stratum Granulosum)
This thin layer provides a waterproof barrier

Transitional Layer

Uppermost Layer of Skin
(Stratum Corneum)
This layer is renewed every 28 days

money is spent to develop them, the moisturizing function of products can't achieve even 1% of our skin's natural moisturizing abilities.

Most man-made products—at best—contain a couple of oils, amino acids, hyaluronic acids, and ceramides. These are no match for the complex substance our body makes for itself. Further, these ingredients in skincare products actually disrupt the body's natural functioning. When you force toners, serums, lotions, or creams onto your skin, you are simply weakening your own powerful, innate moisturizing system and contaminating its hydrating and protective abilities. Using products that have 1% moisturizing ability to substitute our body's own 100% irreplaceable moisturizing machine is just a bad idea, especially when you are damaging that machine at the same time.

Even *if* a product could copy the ingredients and ratio of the body's NMF, products are still far from being able to improve the barrier and moisturizing functions of the skin. Like building a wall, it's not just about having the bricks and mortar; it's about a specific formulation and blend and how they are structurally put together. Would you rather spend your money on a beauty company's damaging imposter or invest your time to learn how to preserve your own powerful, priceless, moisture warrior?

OUR SKIN ARMY

Even though our skin has the ability to protect itself, we cannot forget our mighty helpers: symbiotic microorganisms. They are our army.

The human body is colonized by a diverse milieu of complicated microorganisms, including bacteria, fungi, mites, and viruses. Of those, many have a mutually beneficial relationship with humans. This means both the microbes and the human benefit. Sometimes the relationship is beneficial to the microorganisms, and they do not help or harm the human. This is known as a commensal relationship. When the relationship helps the microbes but harms the human, it is parasitic. Human bodies host all three types of microorganisms, and "symbiotic" refers to the first two types of relationships. Symbiotic microbes find the human body to be a great host on which they can live and feed and form their own community. These communities, called the microbiome, are present in many parts of our body, like in the nose, mouth, gut, vagina, and of course, the skin. These symbiotic microbes live harmoniously on our skin, especially deep in the pores. In exchange, they contribute to us and protect us like a selfish army.

The primary contribution of symbiotic microbes is to occupy space for their own good so that other harmful bacteria and yeast cannot take up residence. They feed on our sebum and sweat (this is one of the reasons these are useful wastes) and produce a slightly acidic substance, known as the acid mantle. The acid mantle is an unwanted substance to pathogens. Harmful bacteria and yeast like to live in an alkaline environment, so the acidic environment makes it difficult for pathogens to reproduce. As long as there are symbiotic microorganisms thriving on our skin, and we are excreting properly, we don't need to worry about losing this acid mantle.

Another contribution of symbiotic microbes is they provide nutrients to the epidermis. Since the epidermis has no blood or lymph vessels, it gets its nutrients via the diffusion of fluids from the dermis, as well as the symbiotic microbes that live in the roots of the hair follicles and sweat glands.[52]

Humans host about a million microorganisms per square centimeter of healthy skin, and there are more microbes in our body than our own cells. The estimated number is in the trillions, with about a thousand different species. Microbiologists have discovered that living creatures rely on microorganisms and their interactions with their hosts for a myriad of life functions: to defend against pathogens, digest food, regulate the immune systems, and germinate seeds. They may even help stabilize our moods and can ward off depression.[53] We don't want to get rid of microbes. Instead, we want to learn to live with them and benefit from them.

These microbes also help educate the immune system—the billions of T cells in the skin—priming it to discriminate between harmless microbes and harmful pathogens.[54] A proper immune response is produced when the body senses true danger from an infection. The immune system kicks into gear and triggers inflammation to attack these invaders, which protects the body and aids healing.[55] However, sometimes an immune system reaction is actually a misfire. This causes significant inflammation and damage to the body's own healthy tissues. Hypersensitivity (allergies) and inflammatory skin disorders are the results of these autoimmune reactions.

We do not know exactly why the skin's immune system misfires and causes hypersensitivity and inflammation (eczema is a good example of this), but we do have plenty of epidemiological data linking frequent and long-term skin product use (especially cleansers) to skin allergies and diseases.

Our skin microbiome forms itself immediately after birth, when bacteria begin to migrate from the mother's birth canal and skin, and colonize the newborn's skin. Capone et al. reported that "the proper microbial colonization of infant skin is crucial and can affect the development of the skin's immune function, the maturation of skin barrier functions, and the body's systemic immune operation."[56] But what do we do to our skin's microbiome from birth? We wash our babies with cleansing products (please understand, whether they are labeled "natural" or "synthetic," the outcome is the same) every day. That causes their skin to become dry, so we smear on moisturizing products to ease the dryness. Both cleansing and moisturizing products contain surfactants, preservatives, fragrances, and additives that change the skin's microbiome, therefore altering the skin's immune functioning.

Right from birth—so early—we begin to wreck the skin.

THE LUSH SKIN GEOGRAPHY

Conventional skin information talks about the stratum corneum as what defines skin beauty because it is positioned on the outermost part of the skin. It is what we see. Scientific literature, however, notes that skin beauty and health go deeper than the stratum corneum. It is the dermatoglyphics, which encompasses multiple layers of skin linked together through metabolic cycles that really defines the skin's beauty and health.

Dermatoglyphics focuses on our skin's geography—a lush land. Under the microscope, healthy dermatoglyphics reveal mesh-like networks of small triangular shapes—an orderly and refined grainy texture as shown in Figure B. The small triangles are plump and hydrated with distinct peaks and valleys, mounds, and grooves to give the skin its elasticity and suppleness. That is the look of healthy skin regardless of age, from babies to elders. Understanding this concept is useful because dermatoglyphics determine the visual status of our skin, not just the structure of the stratum corneum, so it truly impacts what we see. The grains give away how healthy and beautiful the skin is, and this is obvious to the naked eye and verifiable by microscope.

Remember the stratum basale? It is a wavy, intertwining layer between the epidermis and dermis where new cells are generated. The more wavy this juncture, the larger the area for cell regeneration, and the more cells will be made. If the juncture is flat, its total area as well as the number of cells in it will be much fewer. This reduces the number of new cells being produced for the epidermis, which in turn affects the number of cells in the stratum corneum. As a result, the skin will feel tight and pulled, losing its elasticity and suppleness. It becomes shriveled and wrinkled. This is tragic when you realize so much of this damage is self-induced.

If the stratum corneum is disrupted and the moisture barrier is affected, *both* the epidermis and dermis will thin out. The overall skin structure will subsequently thin out. The effect is literally "skin deep"—the *whole skin's depth*. When you use skincare products, you are damaging the stratum corneum, affecting skin regeneration, and reducing the overall quality of your skin. Since the top layer is responsible for regulating all the layers below, it is critical that the top layer be correctly cared for. Once the skin thins, complexion and tone become duller and fine lines become visible. Pigmented blood and lymphatic vessels, nerve fibers, and muscles in the dermis will begin to show through, resulting in spotty skin.

Skincare products that most people in the world believe in are actually harming the top *and* bottom layers of your skin.

FROM THE BEAUTY-OBSESSED SCIENTIST

A SUMMARY AND SOME UTTER BS

I recently saw this commercial: "Nivea Q10 contains natural Q10, 100% identical to the one made by your skin..."

If Nivea's R&D team has the miraculous ability to make "100% identical" substances that our body needs, why haven't they made what the brain, kidneys, pancreas, heart, and joints desperately need so they can cure dementia, glomerulonephritis, diabetes, coronary artery disease, and arthritis? And while they are at it, why not cure cancer as well?

Later in the commercial, they also claim your skin is "as unique as you" and that your skin deserves a unique skin care routine. However, they're advertising this product to every Tom, Dick, and Harriet, and suggesting everyone use it.

So, are we supposed to believe Nivea is tailor-made for each of us even though we also know it is mass-manufactured? Supposedly, this product gives skin "energy and protection, naturally fighting the aging process, and boosting your skin's own anti-aging defense." But if this product is so incredible and powerful, why are there still thousands of products just like it on the market, and why are new ones hitting the shelves all the time?

If skincare products genuinely provided nutrients to our skin, then the skin of those who don't use products would wither and die. We don't see that in babies and kids before they are converted into product users. We also do not see this in adults of nonindustrialized nations where product use is uncommon; nor do we see it in the thousands of clinical cases Dr. Utsugi studied where people stopped using skin products and their skin became healthier. So, the argument that *Skin Sobering* deprives your skin of nutrients just doesn't hold any water or pass any scientific logic. *Skin Sobering* is a process to rid toxins from your skin and certainly does not starve it.

The nutrients and hydration that our skin and body need can only come from within!

Let me summarize Skin 101, repeat several useful terms, and reveal some of the BS out there.

The skin is the largest organ of the body. It is an *excretory* and *protective* organ, so its main functions are to *excrete* waste and create a *barrier* between you and the big, bad world. Any organ that's designed to excrete (poop) does not want to absorb (eat) anything. Exit only! Any organ that is created to protect you doesn't want things to get through it. No penetration!

The skin also wants to exfoliate in order to naturally renew itself. It will shed its dead cells when it is ready so it can *signal* new cells to be made. Further, the skin needs its symbiotic microorganisms to fend off pathogenic ones and to train our immune system to respond appropriately. The skin also helps to regulate the body's internal temperature through sweating while it maintains homeostasis. It is a sensory organ as well, with nerve structures that detect cold, heat, pressure, pain, vibrations, itching, and more.

The skin is quite capable of dealing with nature, *but it is not as equipped to fight off man-made chemicals.* The skin's most vital, overarching function is to preserve its own auto-repairing capabilities. This can only be achieved if the skin's integrity is preserved.

This is just a tidbit of basic physiology and anatomy. When we let modern marketing brainwash us and products grace our skin, we are giving them free rein to disrupt these natural physiological mechanisms. As a result, our skin malfunctions.

CAN THE SKIN ABSORB NUTRIENTS?

As you can see, the skin's many functions are interdependent and interconnected. It serves a variety of protective, homeostatic, sensory, immunological, metabolic, and excretory purposes. But one that has never been mentioned in any scientific literature is the skin's *absorptive and digestive* function! Why? Because that simply isn't how skin functions. It was not designed to eat.

Who told us that the skin has this amazing ability to absorb nutrients? Sales and marketing people, not doctors and scientists. No anatomy or physiology of any mammal's skin is designed to absorb, even though it can. It is meant to be an outlet—just like the urethra! And it's not just chemicals and processed products that your skin will reject: it doesn't want *anything* foreign. So, cucumber slices, avocado paste, honey, lemon, egg whites, and all the other wholesome and organic goodies peddled as skincare substances are *not* welcome on this excretory organ. They are great for your mouth and your digestive system only.

Imagine talking about your anus as a way of "absorbing nutrients" or your urethra as "drinking up moisture" for your body. It would be absurd! Excretory organs and their openings (including skin pores) are made to eliminate wastes. To get nutrients to your skin, you can only go through your mouth.

So when the beauty industry and its beautiful people say that your skin can absorb nutrients fed by their wonderful formulations, they are feeding you utter bullshit!

You may be wondering about suppositories, as they are designed to be inserted through the anus and absorbed by the rectum; catheters, that are inserted into the urethra; or medicated creams and lotions, that are to be absorbed topically. The answer is that suppositories and catheters are for specific medical purposes with the goal of treating an illness, not what our bodies need naturally. Similar to injections that puncture the skin in order to deliver medicine, medicated creams will harm the skin while fulfilling their treatment purpose of delivering medicine. The end justifies the means.

Those medical examples are not evidence that *nutrients* should normally be absorbed this way. Rather, the need for a suppository, an injection, or a catheter is an exception brought on by an illness or malfunction.

That's how we should treat any skin products as well.

For anything to be absorbed *through* the skin, it has to break down and penetrate the skin's "bricks and mortar" first. It must force itself *across* the barrier using chemical or physical action. If you "soak" the skin, sure, it will have to absorb (like a baby's bum absorbing pee from a wet diaper), but that penetration is breaking the skin! Once that happens, your "bricks and mortar" become leaky and TEWL occurs. So you wonder why you feel dry, sensitive, itchy, oily, or have breakouts? Once the skin is weakened and disturbed, your own specific skin weaknesses will worsen.

What about products that claim to be gentle and not break down the skin? Well, if they *don't* break it down, they are not getting in. That means the product just sits on top of your skin, wets your stratum corneum, and fills up your pores. You know what that does to natural exfoliation! The sloughing off of dead cells is also enzymatically controlled,[57] so when the skin is covered with sticky goo, enzymes can't dissolve the bonds holding the corneocytes together, and exfoliation is further hindered. Dead skin cells build up and ugly skin follows.

MOISTURIZATION. EXFOLIATION. SENSITIVITY.

The buildup of dead cells as a result of no natural exfoliation is what makes our skin thick, rough, and dull. We have been fed the idea that we must manually exfoliate this ugly layer away with acids or scrubs. Inevitably, we will remove more layers of dead cells than necessary, causing skin irritation and sensitivity. Exfoliating chemically or mechanically will also aggravate oil gland activity. This increases oil production, causing excessively oily skin. That means acne is soon to follow. All of these problems are created, or at least exacerbated, by using products that we believed would fix these problems. How ironic.

There is a popular Korean product promoter who endorses a "double-cleanse" process and 10-step skin care routine. She has written about chemical and mechanical exfoliation, stating both forms weaken your skin's barrier, so you want to "rehydrate and protect with a good moisturizer."[58] As we know now, this doesn't make sense. Your skin doesn't need any manual exfoliation, but you do it anyway knowing it weakens your skin's barrier? Your skin doesn't need any moisturizer, but you put it on to upset the natural exfoliation. And now you have to put it on after you deliberately exfoliate?

Aren't you creating a new problem while trying to deal with a previous problem you also created?

This particular promoter also asserts that because dead skin cells play an important role in protecting our skin against UV rays and pollutants, a person must use lots of sunscreen after exfoliation. She has some basic knowledge, but the way she pushes products betrays she is a victim of beauty industry brainwashing. Think about ripping off a scab before it's ready to come off on its own—ouch! This is what you are doing to your skin when you manually exfoliate. Of course, sun protection is important, but slathering on irritating chemicals after you just insulted your skin and made it sensitive? This is an example of yet another solution that only creates more and more problems. It is a vicious cycle.

If you have sensitive skin, it means your skin is screaming for help and begging that you stop putting products on it. Unfortunately, beauty-obsessed people are too invested in "helping" their skin to hear its screams.

3

DISBELIEF
WE'VE BEEN LIED TO

EXPOSURE AND BELIEF

A SWEET TALE

SEX SELLS. HOPE AND VARIETY SELL MORE.

DRUGS, TOBACCO, AND ALCOHOL

THE UGLY OLD AUNT WHO DOES NOTHING TO HER SKIN

DO NOTHING EQUALS LOOKING YOUR AGE?

MY "RIDICULOUS" METHOD

DISBELIEVING PATIENTS AND A STUBBORN WIFE

FROM THE BEAUTY-OBSESSED SCIENTIST

We all have some deep-rooted beliefs and ways of doing things. We see these beliefs as "the truth" because they are so familiar to us. To relinquish long-held beliefs about what is good for your skin can be a demanding process of willpower and self-esteem. It really challenges our cognitive ability to see the world differently, especially if the world has been presenting us with a very distorted picture that serves financial agendas rather than the truth.

EXPOSURE AND BELIEF

The more often we hear something, and the more sources we hear it from, the more likely we are to believe it. Social psychologist Robert Zajonc called this the "mere exposure effect," and it is the basis of all successful marketing campaigns.[59] Repeated exposure to something generates cognitive ease. That gives us a sense of psychological safety, and we mistake that safety for truth.

Have you had the experience of hearing a song you didn't much care for at first, but after hearing it over and over you begin to warm up to it? This acceptance is a product of repeated exposure.[60] The tobacco industry heavily participated in this before the '70s with tons of commercials that portrayed smokers as rugged, handsome, physically active, and free.[61,62] The sugar industry is still doing it today, using endless advertisements designed to make us think sugar is wholesome, happy, and rewarding. These commercials convince you that using their products is akin to "being yourself" and "treating yourself" at the same time.

In other words, just do what they say, buy their stuff, and pretend you're doing it for yourself and not for them. Forget about your health consequences while you are at it.

A SWEET TALE

Sugar and skincare products share a similar history of misinformation, a population's misguided beliefs, and hidden dangers. Sugar's danger has been revealed, but the skincare product wolf is still wearing sheep's clothing.

If you think sugar makes your skin bad, you are right. That's one of their connections, but sugar and skincare share something much more alarming: as addicted to sugar as we are, we are equally addicted to skincare products. Worse, just as we were once unaware of the danger and harm associated with increased sugar intake, we have been just as unaware of how harmful skincare products are. Their respective industries successfully kept us in the dark, 蒙在鼓里 (meng zai gu li)—*wrapped inside the darkness of a big drum,* that's worse than an echo chamber. Unfortunately, even now that we are aware of sugar's potential for harm, that harm is still running rampant and wreaking havoc.

For skincare products, we are not even out of the drum.

At the start of the 18th century, the average consumption of sugar in England was roughly 4 pounds per person, per year. That is equivalent to 47 cans of soda per year—less than a can per week. Sugar was a rare treat, and people did not consume enough of it to cause much harm. That number jumped to 22 pounds at the start of the 19th century, over five times the previous amount. Measured in cans of soda, that is 256 cans per year, or 5 cans per week.

Now, in the 21st century, the average North American consumes about 90 pounds of sugar annually. That's about 1,047 cans of Coke a year, or 20 cans a week. That's three cans a day! This number is 20 times higher than the amount consumed three centuries ago, and it has been accompanied by frightening, consequential harm.[63] In the 20th century, we didn't think sugar was bad for our health. We just knew it tasted good, and manufacturers put it in everything. These sugar-added products were marketed with energetic commercials and happy faces. Sugar was no longer a rare treat; it was everywhere. So was obesity, type 2 diabetes, inflammation, heart disease, and fatty liver disease.

The association and the damage are both clear, yet the solution is not easy. People love sugar, and companies sell more food when it contains more sugar. Therefore, companies promote these money-making

DISBELIEF • 53

products with all their might. Clearly, the sugar addiction has gotten worse, and massive amounts of sugary products are made available to us many times a day. Restaurants that swear to not use MSG in their food just replace MSG with sugar. The population is getting sicker, and disease rates have soared across developed countries.

At least we all know this now.

The picture is the same for skincare products, but very few know it yet. We're still being deceived, and it is lasting much longer than the sugary fairy tale did.

Skincare products were nonexistent a couple hundred years ago. Even soap was hard to acquire for most people. When germ theory was popularized in the late 1800s,[64] people learned hygiene and began to wash, primarily with water and basic soap. This practice was very effective in curbing disease transmission and infection. At that time, overall hygiene improved until the advent of the infamous soap opera genre. Remember how soap operas were created to market soap and other skincare products? Just like the exponential growth we saw with sugar and obesity, the severity and prevalence of skin problems exploded too. Childhood eczema soared, beauty issues rose, and sensitivity and dryness skyrocketed.

The more developed the country, the more its people use grooming and skincare products, and the more prevalent skin problems are.

Why did it take so long for us to learn sugar was bad for us? Why can't we see that skincare products are not good for our skin? Many of our incorrect beliefs and the misinformation we've been fed need time to be disproven—time to build evidence and for science to do its work—especially when scientific concepts go against prevailing wisdom or current societal norms.

Imagine trying to explain that the Earth is round during the 16th century, or telling people that smoking is unhealthy and foolish in the 1940s. Imagine attempting to convince parents that baby formula was inferior to breastfeeding in the 1960s, making doctors see that episiotomies should be avoided as a routine birth procedure in the 1970s, or proclaiming that carbohydrates are bad, and fat is fine in the 1980s. You would most likely be deemed a lunatic trying to speak against prevailing wisdom, and good luck getting anyone to listen to you.

So, here we are in 2022 telling you that your skin doesn't need skincare products—natural or synthetic. To some, this may be as outlandish as asking a 16th-century flat Earther to believe the planet is round. Our belief in the (incorrect) prevailing wisdom is so strong, it is easier to think this new skin care information might be wrong. Disbelief that skincare products are bad is not a case of ignorance, nor is it due to a lack of scientific evidence. It is the inescapable noise that the beauty industry has been blasting before our eyes and ears for decades.

How could we *not* believe skincare products are magical when the most beautiful people in the world also tempt us to use them? Why would we ignore the advice of *beauty* professionals and *cosmetic* doctors who tell us our flaws can be reversed if we invest time and money into certain products? Doctors were advertising their favorite brands of cigarettes, and of course doctors were performing routine episiotomies and handing out baby formula. To mess up our brain further, everyone knows "that person," like an aunt, cousin, or friend, who does *nothing* to her skin, and looks old and ugly. This can make us certain that if we don't use products, we will end up looking like an ugly old aunt.

It gets worse. So many people believe there is permanence in the temporary sensations of their skincare products that they protest, "My skin feels best when I use skincare products." These people mistake short-term sensations with long-term results. The repeated use of products simply makes skin worse and worse, with some short periods of looking and feeling better. Usually this comes with a new product, and thus begins the vicious cycle of seeking out newer, better products to secure longer and more lasting effects.

How did sugar dominate the food market, and how does it still reign supreme? How did scientists finally stake their flag in this battlefield, earning a small win by making you understand that refined sugar is bad, but still not succeeding in convincing you to give up sugar? The fight against sugar in the food system is very similar to the fight against skincare products in the beauty world.

Dr. Robert Lustig, a pediatric endocrinologist and professor at the University of California, said in an interview with Dr. Peter Attia that in the North American food system, 10 companies control all consumer-packaged goods and 90% of the calories we consume. Sugar is their business model; the thing that increases sales. When high fructose corn syrup and the dietary guidelines of 1977 ("fat is bad but carbs and sugars are fine") were first available, the profit margin of the food industry increased from 1% to 5% per year. This is their juggernaut, their gravy train. These companies add more sugar and sell more food. Sugar sells, and they know it. That's why there is sugar in virtually all food. Even though the science is incontrovertible that refined sugar is an enemy to our health, food companies are not giving up adding it to almost everything.[65]

Consumers face an impossible, uphill battle when expecting food companies to change the way they do business. This is because companies answer to shareholders, not to consumers. For the sake of public health, the food system needs to change, but they are not going to change it from the inside.

The beauty industry makes for a striking parallel. In the beauty industry, there are *also* 10 companies controlling all the skincare information we receive. We scientists and physicians (the noncosmetic ones) are not able to get the truth to you through the constant marketing barrage of the beauty industry. Health- and beauty-conscious people just want what's good for their skin, yet everything they hear about skin health is falsely connected to product use (sunscreen is an exception and is the lesser of two evils where UV rays are concerned). We are facing an impossible, uphill battle if we expect skincare companies to change the way they do business. They answer to shareholders, not to us, and the claims they make are ultimately designed to bring more money to those shareholders.

The beauty world needs to change, but like the food industry, it is not going to change from the inside. Why? Because selling hope and variety is a wildly successful business model.

SEX SELLS. HOPE AND VARIETY SELL MORE.

Skincare and beauty companies introduce new products every month. They tap into the variety of organic, clean, vegan, non-GMO, responsibly sourced, or something-infused, something-innovative—anything to get you tempted and hopeful. Variety sells more products, and they know it. That's why each company offers so many brands and variants. L'Oréal sells L'Oréal Paris, Garnier, Maybelline New York, SoftSheen, Lancôme, Giorgio Armani, Yves Saint Laurent, and Kiehl's. In fact, L'Oréal sells over 500 brands and thousands of products just for skin.[66]

That is *one* company.

There are nine more giant beauty enterprises whose individual annual revenue is in the hundreds of *billions*. In addition, 20 and counting slightly smaller conglomerates also making billions in sales, and countless small pawns saturate the niche markets, performing cutthroat market grabs using horizontal, vertical,[67] and any other directional segmentation strategy. How many beauty products do you think they collectively put out in the market just in your neighborhood stores? When they throw more products at us, we buy more.

Trying to change the skin and beauty industry is a battle royale, not dissimilar from the tobacco war. You would think health and science had won that one long ago, but the battle against tobacco is still raging on as it tries to rebrand itself with e-cigarettes and vaping.

How likely are we, a physician and a beauty-obsessed scientist, to successfully win against the multibillion-dollar beauty industry? Are we even able to start a skirmish when consumers have been given complex beliefs and misconceptions? After all, we've inherited some of our beauty beliefs from generations who came before our own. It is important to remember that they too suffered from advertising and mixed marketing messages.

It's not just what our mother or grandmother might have told us. It's also the celebrities we love, like Aniston, Jolie, DeGeneres, Vergara, Mirren, Gardner, Washington, Virtue, Paltrow, and more. We love their work and covet their beauty, so why wouldn't we trust what they're endorsing and selling to us?

Let's look at it this way. Are the products really what made these celebrities beautiful? The truth is, they were already beautiful before they used the products. That's one of the reasons they are in show business to begin with. Their beauty is a piece of art and further enhanced (and produced) by makeup, lights, cameras, Photoshop, and a team of talented professionals.

These beautiful people are also paid big bucks to recommend these products, which is fair-market behavior. The celebrities themselves may have been sold a bill of goods they honestly believe in as well. To paraphrase Nassim Taleb, author of *Skin in the Game*, "You can sell me something or you can give me advice, but it's unethical for you to do both."

So why should you believe all that the celebrities say and take their *advice* when you know it's all about them making a profit? Conversely, *Skin Sobering* has nothing to gain, whether you buy or don't buy products in the future. Book sales is our mode of knowledge dissemination, and any profit we might make is minuscule compared to selling skincare products. Our bottom line is people's skin health and beauty.

I want to give these beautiful people my book to convince them that to keep their beauty and to truly promote healthy skin for others, they need *Skin Sobering*.

DRUGS, TOBACCO, AND ALCOHOL

We use the "sobering" concept for skincare products as a way to draw a vivid comparison with alcohol, tobacco, and drugs. Like these substances, skincare products offer a quick and shallow boost. You may feel more "high" and more attractive for a brief time, but all of these "hits" create cumulative harm.

Unfortunately, the public suffers from an *almost total lack of awareness* about the harm that skincare products can cause. Although not as severe or well-known as that of drugs or even sugar, the use of skincare products is much more widespread. The majority of people today still trust that skincare products are nutrients for the skin, primarily just because skincare companies say so. Because of this, we use them under a totally wrong premise. We incorrectly believe that using them is a healthy practice that a responsible person should not neglect. Therefore, we use them way more than other addictive substances—24/7, almost 365. We have been made to believe beautiful skin can only be achieved with products. That's successful marketing—successful brainwashing!

THE UGLY OLD AUNT WHO DOES NOTHING TO HER SKIN

You may have heard many examples that come from the opposite ends of the spectrum like, "I have an aunt who does nothing to her skin, and she looks old and ugly." Or, "My husband doesn't moisturize his skin, and it looks wrinkled and leathery." Or the typical, "My friend is very diligent with her skin care routine, and she looks beautiful." How can we make scientific sense of all this? Are these examples a way to disprove the *Skin Sobering* theory?

When people provide polarized evidence, the listener tends to look at only the circumstances provided: Person A uses nothing, and their skin looks terrible. Person B uses a lot, and their skin looks great. The verdict is crystal clear: product use must be the reason for good skin.

What's missing here? A ton! What else does your aunt or your husband do? Do they expose their face to strong UV rays? Do they smoke or drink? Do they wash their face with cleansers or worse, shampoo that drips down their face, for decades? Do they scrub and rub their skin like they're mopping a dirty floor? Do they eat poorly, have bad sleep habits, or lack exercise? These things combined control a great deal more than the one thing their polarized evidence highlights—that they must be ugly because they don't use skincare products. Without questioning all these confounders, it's too simplistic to just say, "She uses no skincare products, and *that's* the reason she looks terrible."

Conversely, when considering the friend who is diligent with skincare, remember to ask yourself what else is she diligent with? How good is she with all the protection and lifestyle factors mentioned above, and what about the big one: genetics? People who start out looking beautiful tend to do many things, right and wrong, to maintain their beauty. So, what are the real reasons behind their good looks? Is it their other diligent, positive lifestyle habits, and genetics, or is it their dedicated product use?

DO NOTHING EQUALS LOOKING YOUR AGE?

A young actress once said to me, "I don't want to look my age. I want to look younger. If I don't do anything to my skin, won't I just look my own age at best? I'm thirty now. I don't want to look thirty. I will be sixty one day, and I don't want to look sixty. Doing nothing for my skin is expecting it to grow old naturally according to my age. I have no interest in that."

First, not putting products on your skin is *not* "doing nothing" for your skin. It is doing *no harm* to your skin. You are doing a lot for it by *not* harming it. More importantly, what do you think 60-year-old skin *should* look like? What should a 60-year-old person or body look like? Let's use physical health as a comparison, since beauty is so subjective. What should the health of a 60-year-old be? A fit 60-year-old with an active lifestyle may have the health of someone in their 30s. You've seen them. If a person does the right things for their body, it won't show its chronological age. As the person continues to treat her health well, the physical wear and tear that accompanies aging will be much slower. A 70-year-old can have the health of a 35-year-old; 80 can be the new 50. These things are entirely possible.

According to David Sinclair, a professor in the Department of Genetics at Harvard Medical School, aging is a disease, not a normal process.[68] If you do everything right to your body, you will not age in the way you are familiar with, like the mental image of an 80-year-old with a frail, beaten-down body. With proper care and maintenance, your life can extend well past your 80s, even into your 100s, strong and vibrant. What is right for your physical health? Drop smoking and drinking. Avoid sugars, drugs, and processed foods. Eat more plants, get good sleep, and exercise. Our health needs a lot more *harm reduction*, so decreasing harm can give you a level of physical health that makes you look a fraction of your chronological age.

It is not *age* that makes our skin age, but the attacks we put our skin through and the environment it exists in. Putting *nothing* on your skin, as we advocate with *Skin Sobering*, eliminates a massive source of harm. So, stop the attacks—sun damage, bad food, bad life, and skin products—and your skin will look lively and youthful for an enviable length of time. Thirty-year-old skin has the capacity to look as nice as skin in its roaring 20s.

People wrongly assume that putting nothing on their skin means they are doing nothing for it. Putting nothing on your skin reverses harm done to it! When you minimize harm to your skin and health, you will look and feel young for your age.

FROM THE ANTI-AGING DOCTOR

MY "RIDICULOUS" METHOD

I've been told many times that my method is ridiculous. What I am proposing is the complete opposite of what you may have been told, what you've learned, and what you have believed.

That said, the *Skin Sobering* way is really nothing new. The medical field has a long history of advocating using no substances in order to allow the skin to heal and thrive. They just didn't highlight beauty, the most obvious benefit of them all. Our skin regenerates the best when it is left undisturbed and physically protected, especially for common skin beauty issues. I have female and male patients, newborn patients, and patients well into their 80s who started *Skin Sobering* and saw significant improvements. Their skin became healthier and more beautiful with each additional year. Their clinical assessment data provides solid proof.

Regardless of what skin care method one uses, it is not possible to have 100% satisfaction. Some of my patients tried *Skin Sobering* but couldn't persist and quit halfway through. Most of them experienced dryness, and they feared that if they didn't put something back on their skin, it would get worse. Sadly, they did not get through this "withdrawal" stage and were not able to shake their dependence on products.

When you use products, you do experience a quick effect of smoothness and softness. This is especially true for dry and dehydrated skin. You will feel that you have nicer skin *while* the products are on it, just like when you are high on addictive drugs. As soon as the products are off, the feelings of tightness, dryness, pulling, and/or flakiness reappear. And you will feel the need for more products while your skin is slowly but surely deteriorating. With the naked eye, my patients' skin didn't seem to have much damage from the products. However, under the microscope, it's so obvious that their pores had been assaulted by products. At that level, inflammation is everywhere, and people can feel it—in the most benign form of dryness, sensitivity, or the catchall term, aging. When you use skincare products long-term, they become your "skin crack." Without them, you don't feel right.

Why do people continue to use skincare products even though their skin is showing signs of damage? I showed my patients their skin under the microscope and recommended they stop using products for four weeks. Most of them noticed their skin improved, but very few considered quitting skincare products altogether. Instead, they wanted to find different, better, more natural products, and restart using them. Their belief about products (more accurately, product marketing claims) is so ingrained. Back and forth they go, repeating the cycle many times, until they are hurt long enough to finally realize that not using any skincare products (including cleansers) gave them their best skin.

DISBELIEVING PATIENTS AND A STUBBORN WIFE

I deeply understand how difficult it is to challenge and change this indoctrinated belief. I have told many of my patients, "Your skin is the worst kind. It is the most damaged, Type III skin." Most of them were shocked and hurt by my statement. I can empathize. To be told by a specialist that your skin is in severely bad shape, hurts. To find out that all the money, time, and energy you spent on taking care of your skin has actually led to damage feels shameful, bruising your self-esteem. Some of them would reply angrily, "You made me feel like a fool!" But my words are coming from the right place, from an attempt to save your skin: 苦口良藥 (ku kou liang yao)—*good herbal medicine tastes bitter.*

I can no longer, with any conscience, continue to sell products to my patients.

From a very young age, we've been told to take care of our skin with products. To suddenly quit this practice and forgo this belief can be puzzling and difficult. To make matters worse, most people experience dryness when they initially begin *Skin Sobering*. Why is that?

SKIN SOBERING EQUALS DRYNESS?

When our skin's natural protective barrier has been damaged, moisture is the first thing that escapes and dryness soon follows. When you apply lotions or creams on this dry skin, your skin will look moisturized. This is just the "gooey" substance soaking your skin, covering up the leakiness, dryness, and roughness. This is an illusion of hydration. Regrettably, it is creating more leakiness at the same time. As soon as you stop using these products, your skin reverts to feeling dry and rough. The bottom line is that these products are just whitewashing your skin's flaws while slowly eating it up.

Your skin's initial reaction to *Skin Sobering* will unfortunately reveal how bad a shape your skin is truly in—dry, oily, flaking, breaking out—whatever your inherent and induced problems are. Your skin becomes a terrible landscape. This is exactly the withdrawal effect from quitting a drug, a type of "skin crack" that's been giving you temporary pleasure while damaging your body.

MY STUBBORN WIFE

At first, my wife couldn't accept the *Skin Sobering* way. Basically, she just didn't believe me. It was only because her "expert" husband insisted, "It's best for your skin not to use any skincare products," that she unwillingly tried.

For a couple of months, it appeared that she had quit products, but she was actually secretly using them. When I noticed blemishes on her skin, I asked, "Why are you continuing with the products? Can't you see the little bumps?" She contended, "When I don't put anything on my skin, it feels like it's going to peel off. I worry that I'll end up with fine lines and wrinkles! And why is it that besides you, no one else is promoting this kind of skin care?" We fought many times because of this disagreement.

It's true. No one is promoting this kind of skin care, but that is because there's no money to be made. Promotion is married to product sales. Even though there are many scientific studies showing the benefits of no skincare products, no one is promoting them to the general public. I continued to encourage my wife. "Your skin will become more beautiful. Tolerate the process and persist!"

It took Noriko, my wife, two years to completely kick her "skin crack" habits. After her second year of *Skin Sobering*, her dermatoglyphics became bountiful and full again. Today, her skin is healthy and beautiful. She's had "sober skin" for over 10 years now, and she only applies makeup in some small, key areas when needed. She does not use foundation at all.

Noriko recalled, "In the first few months, I struggled tremendously, wondering if this would really work. If it wasn't for your encouragement and addressing my concerns, I would've given up the practice for certain. I think you need to write a book about the harm of products so others can have your reassurance and their questions answered."

Before *Skin Sobering*, Noriko would buy all sorts of skincare products, especially when she traveled. These expensive bottles would fill her vanity counter. Now there's nothing on her counter. She thanks me often for her beautiful skin and for her simple skincare routine. And I am grateful for my happy and beautiful wife!

Those who start *Skin Sobering* are bound to see some initially undesirable changes in their skin. This will be your weakest time, when you are most likely to fall for the temptation of using products again. Your disbelief will creep back in. How do you gain the strength to persist? Understand how your skin is made and what products are made of. You need to power your determination with facts and science.

4

(BIO)CHEMISTRY
PRODUCTS THAT CLAIM TO HEAL US ARE HURTING US

OILS AND SURFACTANTS

MOISTURIZERS DRY OUR SKIN—IRONIC?

NATURAL OILS AND THE
OIL-SUNNING PHENOMENON

PRESERVATIVES AND GERMS

CLEANSING PRODUCTS REMOVE MORE THAN YOU WANT

THE HARM OF SCRUB AND RUB

WATER IS NOT *ALL* WONDERFUL

FROM THE ANTI-AGING DOCTOR

Now that you know the structures and functions of the skin, let's look at what skincare products do to it.

No matter how expensive your skincare product is, it is inferior to your body's own NMF. Skincare products are really just a mixture of contaminants, yet so many people still believe the opposite. They continue to care for their skin with products and thus render their skin into a problematic state. Then they blame—and marketing messages have taught them to blame—these problems on aging. In this chapter, we will specifically discuss how skincare products burden and damage the skin.

OILS AND SURFACTANTS

Let's first understand our own oil, known as sebum.

Sebum is a mixture of oils and fats secreted by the sebaceous (oil) glands.[69] These glands usually open into a hair follicle, and the secreted, oily, waxy matter lubricates the hair and the skin (see Figure D in Chapter 2). Sebaceous glands are distributed over the entire body, with the exception of our palms and soles. They are most plentiful on the scalp and face, but they are also found in hairless areas like the eyelids, nose, penis, and labia minora. Another type of gland is the sweat gland. As the name implies, it secretes sweat, which is watery in nature. Sweat glands are important for controlling the temperature of the body and for excreting waste products.[70]

There are two kinds of sweat glands: eccrine and apocrine. Eccrine glands are distributed all over the body and mainly secrete water and electrolytes, which don't smell. Apocrine glands are larger and also open into the hair follicle. They are also abundant in your armpits and groin, and they secrete a fatty sweat. The fats attract bacteria, which break them down into smelly, fatty acids. These glands and follicle openings are the infamous pores commercials tell us we must work to shrink.

Sebum forms the slightly greasy surface film of the skin and helps to keep it flexible. However, excessive sebum is not good for the skin. Sebum oxidizes when exposed to outside elements, such as UV rays and pollutants. This oxidative reaction turns sebum into *squalene peroxide*, which can cause inflammatory damage to the skin.

"We must wash [the sebum] off thoroughly. Once the skin is fully cleansed, then we must moisturize it with lotion, cream, or oil, to restore the skin's moisture!" You have heard different versions of the above countless times from skincare companies. They claim to use science, but they twist the information for their marketing purposes.

If your skin's own oil can oxidize, what do you think happens with the processed oils you put on your skin? Again, remember that it does not matter whether the product claims to be natural or synthetic. These lotions and creams are worse than your natural sebum because of the other necessary ingredients in them: preservatives, fragrances, additives, and *surfactants*. This last category of compounds is relatively unknown to the public, but is most ubiquitously used in products.

SURFACTANTS

Surfactants[71] are compounds that lower the surface tension between two substances, just like an emulsifier. They have both hydrophilic (water-loving) and lipophilic (lipid-loving) properties, so they are referred to as *amphiphilic*.[72] Lotions and creams are made up of a mixture of oil and water. Oil and water don't mix, but with the addition of surfactants, the two can mingle smoothly together. Natural emulsifiers or surfactants are used in the food world all the time. They make salad dressings smooth and ice creams creamy. Besides being used in lotions and creams, surfactants are in cleansers, serums, shampoos, conditioners, detergents—essentially anything that's in a liquid or viscous form.

As stated in Chapter 2, the stratum corneum is made up of a neatly stacked, brick-like wall of corneocytes and mortar-like, intercellular substances. Corneocytes are filled with water-soluble (hydrophilic) amino acids, and the intercellular substances contain fat-soluble (lipophilic) ceramides, cholesterol, and fatty acids. Together, they make up the NMF,[73] with its incredible moisture-retaining ability. This dual formation gives the skin a tough yet supple, hydrated barrier that can resist environmental assaults.

However, lotions, creams, and the extended family of "caring" products can quickly and easily damage the human body's remarkable moisture barrier because of surfactants (as well as other substances in the products). The amphiphilic abilities of surfactants can dissolve the water-based contents of the corneocytes and the oil-based bonds of the intercellular substances, eat up the bricks-and-mortar wall, the NMF, and eventually destroy the stratum corneum's structure—not in one day, but day after day. The skin's moisture retainer and barrier, no matter how incredible and strong, will have little chance of functioning well if the skin is being loaded up with products daily, for years and decades.

If you continue using products, your skin's natural and wondrous abilities won't have a chance against the chemicals. Once your skin is weakened, water and moisture will leak. Your skin is no longer an intact barrier, and many more bad things can happen to it.

MOISTURIZERS DRY OUR SKIN—IRONIC?

Besides surfactants, many skincare products also have "miracle active ingredients" meant to help accelerate the improvement of your skin. The oils, surfactants, and numerous active ingredients have the ability to seep into your skin through your pores and slowly dissolve your moisture barrier. The chemical names and claimed functions of these active ingredients change from brand to brand, season after season, so it's a fool's game to try to name them or keep up with them. These substances, just like sebum, oxidize and become rancid even faster. The pores and skin tissues *know* these substances are foreign to them, so the skin rejects them, manifesting its dismay quietly in the form of inflammation.

When pores and tissues become inflamed, they try to heal, as skin naturally wants to do. If products are continuously applied to the skin, the pores and tissues inflame again. They get into another battle to heal and inflame. The cycle repeats, and the condition becomes chronic. This frequent recurrence stimulates melanin precipitation, which causes the skin to be blotchy and hyperpigmented. As this cycle continues, dark spots and dullness become chronic also. Dryness is not the only problem that accompanies lotions and creams.

When I examined my product-loving patients' skin under the microscope, I saw inflammation around almost all of their pores. In the more severe cases, their pores were shaped like a volcanic pothole, with swelling all around the circumference. The collagen that's holding up the dermis is being dissolved by these "miracle" products too, which are now truly penetrating deep inside, affecting not just the epidermis but the dermis as well. Why does damaged skin sag? Because the skin's deeper layers are also impacted over time.

In dermatology, the intended purpose of lotions and creams is to *disrupt* the protective barrier of the skin so *medicinal* drugs can penetrate the skin to heal something. Creams are the most powerful, then lotions, then gels. Because these substances can disrupt the skin's barrier in such an effective way, they have irritating and inflammatory side effects. Therefore, the treatment benefits of the medicine must be much greater than the harm of the carrier (the cream) for this damage to be worth it. Again, the end justifies the means.

Yet, the purpose of most skincare products is not to treat an illness. They are advertised to make skin beauty issues appear better. Why should we allow them to harm our skin by causing irritation and inflammation while at the same time *inducing* more skin beauty problems? They are not like medicinal ointments, which you are instructed to use sparingly and for a limited period of time. These skincare products are marketed to be applied day and night—till death do you part!

Do they really improve your skin and protect it against deterioration? The answer, of course, is no.

NATURAL OILS AND THE OIL-SUNNING PHENOMENON

"What about the natural oils: camellia, jojoba, olive, coconut, shea butter, squalene, lanolin, lavender, lemon, eucalyptus, tea tree, peppermint, jasmine, ylang ylang, and so on—all those beautiful-sounding, pure, essential oils? They don't contain any surfactants, so I don't have to worry about them like I do with lotions and creams, right? They must be good for the skin, right?"

Unfortunately, natural oils are no better than synthetic or organic lotions and creams. These oils are lipophilic, so they can dissolve fats and oils. These oils will get into the fatty, intercellular substance—the "mortar" space. Since they are foreign objects and irritants to the skin, your skin tissue will fight and repel them, resulting in inflammation. If used frequently and liberally, these oils can directly dissolve the whole intercellular mortar. Your moisture barrier is now defective and your skin is at risk of being dehydrated, all from having moisturizing oil on it!

The long-term use of oils can lead to another skin problem, one that causes hyperpigmentation, like the sun does. The Asian cosmetic world calls this the "oil-sunning phenomenon." How does this happen? When you use oil on your skin daily, your skin will shrink and become thinner. Why? As we discussed in Chapter 2, the stratum basale generates new cells only when signals from the stratum corneum are sent down. This occurs when the corneocyte dead cells naturally flake off. Essential oils, or other skincare products that contain oil, will make the skin sticky and gooey, thus preventing dead skin cells from flaking off. No signal is sent down, and very few new cells are made. The stratum corneum becomes thick and coarse from dead cells not falling off, and the epidermis gets thin and old from new cells not being made.

How can your skin look good when it is going through this?

Further, oils oxidize when exposed to air. These oxides (which are free radicals) are also unwanted irritants to the skin, so the skin inflames in order to fight them. Once this inflammation turns chronic, it will induce blotchy pigment production and cause your skin to lose its glow. Now the skin looks even worse: dull pigment from inflammation, a coarse stratum corneum, and a thin epidermis that shows more spots. This is just like sun-damaged skin.

We hope this new knowledge makes you think twice about putting essential oils on your skin. If you use essential oils for their smell, then dab some in hidden skin parts you don't mind damaging or, even better, in a few strands of hair. Hair is good for retaining scent.

PRESERVATIVES AND GERMS

The health of our skin depends on symbiotic microorganisms and their microbiome.

We did a microbes count on the faces of staff members at the Research Centre. I had no history of habitual skincare product use, and there were about 600,000 symbiotic microorganisms on a small oily area of my skin. The same count was done on my nurses and female staff, who were skincare product users, and there were hardly any of these beneficial microbes on their face. One woman had less than 500! The one with the highest count had merely 30,000, an insignificant number compared to healthy skin. The microbiome almost didn't exist on their faces. Why did they have so few good microbes in this ecosystem? How were skincare products impacting this?

Plastic surgeons are using fewer and fewer disinfectants to clean the skin and wounds to preserve the skin's natural healing abilities. If we didn't cover the disinfectant bottles well, bacteria would grow in the solution after a few weeks. It would become muddy and spoiled.

I stress, I am talking about bottles filled with *disinfectants*!

Yet toners, lotions, foundations, and most types of skin products can be left for years without going bad because of added preservatives. The microorganism-killing power of these preservatives is even stronger than surgical disinfectants! Very few microbes have a chance to survive in them.

Yet our body needs these microbes. When these strong preservatives are applied to the face day after day, you can bet most of the symbiotic microbes are destroyed. They may have a chance to live if there's only one product attacking them, but most people—particularly women—apply layer after layer of multiple products on their face. What's the fate of their microbiome? When you use two products, you double the amount of preservatives on your skin. With three products, preservatives triple.

You get the arithmetic. Korean skin care routines recommend a 10-step, 10-product practice. They sell 10 times the products, and you get 10 times the assault. Who's the benefactor here, and who's the sucker?

Another frightening finding from multiple product users was that some *invasive* germs had begun to take over. This pathogenic germ is *Malassezia*, a form of yeast that grows in the sebaceous areas of the skin, such as the scalp, brows, and nose. Malassezia can proliferate rapidly when your skin army is destroyed and when the preservatives (destructive in their own right) are no longer on your skin to kill everything, for better or for worse. With your army gone, your skin must rely on preservatives and other harmful chemicals to kill bad pathogens. In this rare period of a temporary off-balance 青黄不接 (qing huang bu jie)—*the growing, green crop can't catch up to the depleting, yellow reserves*—you may get seborrheic dermatitis. It is also known as eczema and psoriasis, a prevalent condition in modern society, especially in young children. If the skin's microbes are living in healthy equilibrium, and symbiotic ones are back to good numbers, pathogenic yeasts will have a hard time occupying the skin.

I often joke, "If someone is really into cleansing, skin care, and makeup, don't get near their skin. It's full of terrifying germs."

CLEANSING PRODUCTS REMOVE MORE THAN YOU WANT

We have talked about the harm of skincare products, but most people are unaware that cleansers and makeup removers belong to that group as well. Cleansing is an integral part of almost every skincare routine, but cleansing with products is even more problematic for your skin—with one saving grace.

There are many types of cleansers and makeup removers—oils, lotions, gels, foam, milk, micellar water, and new ones we can't keep up with. An important ingredient in all of these removers and cleansers is *surfactant*—the same culprit. Makeup removers are the worst of them all, with the ability to remove the most stubborn oil-based makeups. While the makeup is being removed, so is your skin's precious acid mantel, microbiome, and NMF—really, your entire moisture barrier. The surfactants in makeup removers will dissolve both the lipid-soluble and water-soluble substances, along with whatever microorganisms exist naturally on your skin.

Makeup removers possess such superb stripping power because of the high quantity of surfactants in them. This amount much exceeds what's in cleansers, creams, and lotions. Once you use makeup remover, no residue of makeup is left. You are happy about that, because that's what you've been told to achieve—no trace of makeup—but there *is* something left on your skin: a lot of harmful surfactants. Now, you must wash off these surfactants with cleansers, but what is in cleansers? Again, surfactants, preservatives, additives, and so on. Your skin is taking a continual beating!

As surfactants dissolve your skin's moisture barrier, your natural protective ability starts to weaken. When the moisture barriers are disrupted, it takes at least three to four days for them to regenerate and repair, and that is if you leave them alone. However, if you use removers, cleansers, or any "leave-on" products (I realize this encompasses almost all skincare products) again before the repair is done, you are adding insult to injury, further disturbing your skin's recovery. The Chinese have a similar saying: 傷口撒鹽 (shang kou sa yan)—*sprinkle salt on the wound*. If you continue the damage using even mild chemical cleansers to clean your skin every day and night, you will lose your natural protection. No expensive or plant-based moisturizers can rebuild your skin's own natural protective, moisturizing functions.

Compared to smearing on skincare products, cleansing with products assaults the skin much more. The one saving grace? If you remove the cleanser right after cleaning, the strong, harmful action is only present on your skin for a few minutes. Skincare products people leave on, however, stick around to damage the skin. Which is worse? There's no point in comparing. There's no lesser evil here.

When removers and cleansers scrape off the skin's protective barriers, the skin quickly loses inner moisture and oil. Significant dehydration and dryness sets in, and the skin shrivels and atrophies. It can no longer fulfill its job of flaking and sending signals, causing the metabolic mechanism of cell turnover and skin renewal to break down.

The natural result of using makeup removers and cleansers is dryness and tightness. What do people do to address this unpleasant outcome? They apply skincare products to "replenish" moisture and to make the skin feel okay again. This chemical answer is short-lived. The harmful ingredients in skincare products can seep deep into damaged skin, destroying the composition of the moisture barrier even further. That's why so many people experience redness, itchiness, dryness, inflammation, and sensitivity—these are not part of life, nor normal feelings of skin. The skin's miraculous recovering power can't withstand these constant attacks. Your skin turns dull, loses elasticity, and becomes thin, wrinkly, and saggy. Your skin looks beaten and old—not from age itself, but from the products with which it has been assaulted.

NEXT COMES THE DISEASE

Overcleansing with products does not only lead to minor beauty problems like dryness, sensitivity, and enlarged pores. It can also cause seborrheic dermatitis (this time unrelated to Malassezia). When your natural oil is chemically washed off, the skin defends itself by producing more. The overproduction of oil can lead to this form of dermatitis, which is characterized by flakes, redness, and itchiness. This can be especially prevalent in the oily parts of the face, like the sides of the nose, eyebrows, ears, eyelids, and chest. The oil glands get larger from overproduction, and the pores protrude and enlarge at the same time. As the problem persists, the skin takes on an orange-peel texture—pitted, dimpled, and puckered. The overworked glands make the skin oilier and rougher but do not help with dehydration. This layers a new problem on top of any old problems.

In those with sensitive skin, almost every pore on their skin is inflamed. Our naked eye may not see that, but these puffy pores can go from being red and inflamed to becoming dark and swollen, not unlike the bumpy craters on the moon. *Three feet of ice did not come from one day's cold* 冰凍三尺非一日之寒 (bing dong san chi fei yi ri zhi han). In other words, this level of inflammation is not the result of a few days of doing the wrong thing. It's from daily and long-term product use.

THE HARM OF SCRUB AND RUB

Another damaging consequence from these makeup removers is the scrubbing and rubbing that comes with the territory. To dissolve and remove all the makeup, most people will rub the remover into their skin, then wipe the mixture off, stretching the skin while they are at it. These rub, scrub, wipe, stretch actions, and the surfactants in skincare products, are all adding fuel to the fire. Your NMF is like the slime on an eel's skin, and it protects the skin from getting dry. For the eel, if that layer of slime is scrubbed away, its skin will dry up and it will die. Similarly, if our skin's NMF is scrubbed off, our skin will dry up, but we don't die. Our skin will just wither.

Every time the NMF is removed, it takes three to four days for it to be replenished. This is the case even for healthy skin. For most people who use products, their NMF is further depleted, and it will take much, much longer than a few days for their skin to return to its pre-distressed state. Under this product-covered condition, NMF cannot regenerate timely. It simply can't catch up, and this leaves the skin in a chronic state of lacking natural moisture. Slowly and steadily, as cell regeneration also ceases, this unhealthy skin will thin out, wrinkle, and sag. At that point, your skin doesn't just look bad under the microscope—it looks horrible to the naked eye!

Rubbing and scrubbing will also lead to inflammation. This stimulates melanocyte cells and causes patchy dark spots and dullness. If the rubbing and scrubbing doesn't stop, the tough stratum corneum will multiply quickly to protect the skin from further physical pressure, similar to when calluses form on your heels or palms. This defensive growth will cause dead skin on your face to thicken, mimicking the look of unsightly, callused heels.

How ironic! Skincare products and the physical actions needed to apply and remove them cause the skin to be dry, pigmented, thin, and thick in all the wrong places. Your skin's visible age is not a result of you growing old. Rather, it is a reflection of the way you treat it and the products—or lack of products—you use!

WATER IS NOT *ALL* WONDERFUL

When you read that water is problematic for your skin, you might be surprised. After all, the *Skin Sobering* way is all about water. You hear about the wonders of water everywhere, from magazines, TV ads, aestheticians, and friends. They all say that having moisture or water *on* your skin is the most important part of keeping it moisturized.

On the contrary, the proof that water is not good for the skin's *surface* is everywhere in daily life.

When our face or hands are covered with water, our instinctive reaction is to wipe it off. The reason is water can disrupt the protective function of the skin. Your skin has the ability to prevent water from evaporating from *underneath* it, and it can block foreign substances. If there is water residue on top of our skin long enough, the skin's barrier can be altered. Humans know this fact intuitively, which is why even babies and young kids instinctively wipe water off their faces. You may not have consciously thought about this, so try it tonight. Wash your face, but only dry your hands and leave your face wet. See how long you can stand it. Swimming or taking a bath immerses the entire body in water, so it is different from leaving water on the face when everywhere else is dry. Even when you are swimming, you wipe water off your face as soon as you come up for air. Water is essential, but it isn't good to let it sit on the surface of your skin for prolonged periods of time.

So, how does water harm the surface of the skin?

Whether it is toner, lotion, or water, none of them have the ability to moisturize the skin from the outside. Not only that, they all dry out the skin. The NMF that our skin produces is totally different from water. It is a complex combination of amino acids, fatty acids, and electrolytes. These perfectly balanced substances *retain* water *within* the skin and prevent *evaporation*. Yet lotions and toners are mainly made up of water. Water not only doesn't moisturize the skin, but it evaporates. When water evaporates from the skin, the skin behaves like a wet newspaper being air-dried: the top layer will wrinkle, warp, curl, and lift off from the layer underneath (*not* natural exfoliation, which is a different story). The longer this evaporation process continues, the more layers will warp and lift, resulting in a multilayer peeling. This is the stratum corneum layer, the skin's top layer, sustaining the first degree of damage.

When these outermost top layers warp and curl up, cracks form between the corneocyte "brick" cells. The moisture that was protected by the wall of "bricks and mortar" can now slowly leak out and evaporate through the cracks. This makes the skin more dry. Toners and lotions not only *cannot* moisturize your skin, but they actually cause it to dry out.

Some skincare methods actually promote leaving your skin wet for a few minutes to make your skin soft and smooth. There is no scientific basis for this suggestion.

IT'S NOT JUST WATER.
MY PREMIUM PRODUCTS HAVE ACTIVE INGREDIENTS.

"But it's not just water in these lotions! My products contain hyaluronic acids and other wonderful hydra-plumping ingredients that possess great moisturizing abilities!" People who have some skin care knowledge may quickly reach for this rebuttal.

This is a big misunderstanding.

Water makes up 90% of the content in skincare products. Besides surfactants, preservatives, and fragrances, many lotions also contain hyaluronic acids, ceramide, vitamin C, collagen, and other pricy proteins and vitamins. These substances have good moisturizing abilities *when they exist natively within our skin*. So, these skincare products should have good moisturizing functions, right?

I regret to tell you, the answer is no. These added substances actually dry out skin even more than water.

Water evaporates quite quickly when it is sitting on your skin. However, if there are additives like hyaluronic acids and collagen present, as they are in lotions and moisturizers, it will take longer for the water to evaporate. This is because the substance is more viscous. The longer water remains on the surface of the skin, the more cell layers will warp and lift, and the more moisture will be lost. So, the exact same amount of water will cause more damage to your skin if it takes eight hours to completely evaporate as opposed to eight minutes. The stratum corneum cells will deform and crack more severely when the evaporation process takes more time, and this leaves the skin more damaged.

Even worse, once the water has evaporated out of the lotion, the remaining dried hyaluronic acid and collagens will turn powdery. This powdery residue just sits on the skin and will induce further evaporation and damage. Instead of keeping the skin moist, these precious active ingredients that you've possibly even paid more for actually suck up more water from deep within your skin, dehydrating it further.

Why is this happening? Hyaluronic acid and collagen are solids, which need to be ground into powder before they can be added to skincare products. Once powders dissolve in lotions and creams, they become thicker. Think about adding cornstarch to water when you're cooking. This thickens the liquid and turns it into a paste. The paste can evaporate, returning the cornstarch to its floury, powder form. Water in these thickened lotions and creams evaporates just the same, obeying the laws of physics. After six to eight hours of being on the skin, the hyaluronic acid and collagens will turn back into their original powdered form. We know powder facilitates evaporation, causing any water on the skin's surface to evaporate more (like using talcum powder on a baby's bum or for treating heat rash in the old days). When the skin's surface is already dry, the powder residue goes deeper and steals more moisture from deep underneath your skin.

The sales pitch that these products "lock in moisture" is not only fake, but it's the complete opposite of what actually happens to your skin. Instead of locking in moisture, these products trap your skin in a dry prison, stripping away more and more of your skin's natural moisture.

"But," some may say, "my skin is so hydrated when I use skincare products, especially the rich and luxurious ones."

The hydrated look indeed comes from those eight hours (some products claim to last 48 hours) of *delayed* evaporation. So, the more ingredients you put in the products, the longer water is trapped on the surface of the skin by these powdery additives. Your skin looks smooth and plump when water is there. As soon as the water is gone—which the laws of chemistry and physics assure us it will be—your skin will become even more cracked and dry. It will desperately crave another fix of "skin crack" to look plump and beautiful again.

Sounds like these expensive active ingredient additives are a lot like drugs!

Hyaluronic acid and collagen naturally exist in our skin. They have the critical job of keeping our skin supple and moist *from within*. This is why people have the impression that these agents are good for our skin. They are, but not when applied from *outside*! However, because they have the ability to make our skin feel moist, they are popular. Remember, expensive-sounding ingredients serve the purpose of elevating brand image. They do *not* help your skin!

5

DAMAGE

HOW DOES OUR BODY INCUR AND RESPOND TO DAMAGE?

INFLAMMATION AND HEALING

CHRONIC INFLAMMATION
AND SKIN CONDITIONS

ALLOW YOUR IMMUNE RESPONSE TO HEAL YOU

INFLAMM-AGING

INVISIBLE INFLAMMATION, SKIN SENSITIVITY,
AND THE DISEASE EPIDEMIC

FROM THE BEAUTY-OBSESSED SCIENTIST

There is increasing evidence that inflammation is an underlying physiological process of many chronic illnesses and skin problems.[74] Everything from diabetes, metabolic syndrome, cancer, cardiovascular disease, rheumatoid arthritis, inflammatory bowel disease, asthma, and chronic obstructive lung disease to skin irritation, itchiness, redness, puffiness, blemishes, flakiness, hyperpigmentation, acne, dullness, sensitivity, and more can all be attributed to inflammation.[75]

INFLAMMATION AND HEALING

Inflammation is the body's normal healing mechanism. It is a biological defense process where the immune system recognizes things that harm it, such as infections, injuries, and toxins.[76] It responds by releasing antibodies and proteins and increasing blood flow to the damaged area. This process is meant to remove harmful and foreign stimuli. The body then begins to heal. When you scrape your knee, your antibodies and proteins clot your blood and reduce blood flow, your immune system ramps up, and inflammation occurs.[77] This inflammation is normal and necessary for healing. Your antibodies also eat the dead skin cells and germs around the injured area. Once the wound is free of germs and foreign bodies, new skin starts to grow, and the antibodies leave. It is crucial that these antibodies leave, because having continual inflammation can lead to serious problems.

Inflammation can be either acute or chronic. With acute inflammation, where tissues are often damaged, inflammation starts rapidly, becomes severe quickly, and then subsides in a few days after the foreign stimuli or infections are cleared. Acute inflammation usually causes noticeable symptoms, such as pain, redness, or swelling.[78] However, chronic inflammation symptoms are more subtle. This also means they are easily overlooked, especially on your skin.

CHRONIC INFLAMMATION AND SKIN CONDITIONS

Chronic inflammation is slow and can last for a period of months to years.[79] In the case of skin health, chronic inflammation happens when foreign irritants continue to exist on the skin, and/or when the immune response is faulty, leaving the skin in a constant state of alert. Irritation causes inflammation immediately, whether you can see it or not, and damage takes place even though the skin may not show it right away.[80]

The most common manifestation of chronic inflammation of your skin is sensitivity. Other symptoms are itchiness, redness, puffiness, hyperpigmentation, blemishes, flakiness, acne, dullness, and even wrinkles. These have too often been viewed as just beauty issues, or worse, a "natural" part of aging. Yet they are as real and as deserving of proper care as any other inflammation in our body.

ALLOW YOUR IMMUNE RESPONSE TO HEAL YOU

There is a difference between *infection* and *inflammation*.[81] Infection refers to the invasion and proliferation of a pathogen within the body, while inflammation is the body's defensive response against infection. When it comes to the skin, an inflamed site doesn't necessarily mean your skin needs drugs or topical substances to heal the area. These substances usually interfere with your immune system's healing mechanism and render the inflammation worse. Unless the substance's benefits outweigh its harm, don't rush to apply anything to your skin.

Don't be afraid of your skin getting red and swelling during the first few days of a recovery stage—again, this is part of normal healing. Keep your inflamed site clean with water and pure soap, and observe and understand how your body responds. When your skin is infected, it means the pathogens present have grown large enough in number that your immune system is having a hard time fending them off. That is when you need outside help. It is very important to know when to interfere and when to let time do its work. Learning about your body can give you that distinguishing ability.

When you get a little cut or a zit, and it starts looking a bit red and swollen the next day, don't put products on it right away. That swelling is your immune system working, and inflammation is part of the healing process. Clean the site thoroughly with soap and water, or a quick, targeted application of rubbing alcohol twice daily. Left alone and carefully cleaned, your skin will heal in three to four days. However, if you don't keep it clean, or if your immune response is compromised, and the inflammation worsens into an infection, you will need to treat it with medicine. Otherwise, don't disturb your skin with products and cause further irritation. Allow it to heal naturally. That's the best form of healing with the lowest risk of scarring, and the best training for your immune system and future cell regeneration.

INFLAMM-AGING

Inflammation has such a profound effect on skin health that medical literature has a term for it—"Inflamm-aging." Inflamm-aging points to chronic, low-grade inflammation that is believed to accelerate aging and worsens many age-related conditions. Chronic inflammation, acute inflammation, and irritation of the skin can all destroy its protective barrier and integrity. Over time, inflammation impairs the skin's immune and repair responses, damaging its collagen and elastin components. With a weakened barrier, pathogens can enter more easily, increasing the risk of skin breakouts. So, the classic inflammatory symptoms of pain, redness, and swelling may not plague your face, but if inflammation continues, the common beauty issues of dryness, sensitivity, itchiness, wrinkles, sagginess, and scarring will rear their ugly heads sooner or later. Just *how* ugly these will look depends on your body's ability to repair the damage.

INVISIBLE INFLAMMATION, SKIN SENSITIVITY, AND THE DISEASE EPIDEMIC

When it comes to skin sensitivity, 9 times out of 10, invisible inflammation and preexisting conditions are the true culprits.[82] Some literature attributes a compromised barrier function as the origin and the cause of inflammation. A barrier with cracks in it will permit unwanted agents to get in, causing inflammation, moisture leakage, subsequent dryness, and signs of aging.

But is the compromised barrier function the *origin* and *cause* of inflammation, or is it the *result* and *effect* of something else?

We were not born with a leaky stratum corneum. Our protective barrier becomes leaky as a result of environmental and chemical attacks. These attacks are the cause of so many skin issues. Sensitive skin is a consequence of our modern society's way of cleansing and caring for our skin. This explains the increasing prevalence of skin reactions and diseases in industrialized societies.

Invisible inflammation is responsible for skin sensitivity and the skin disease epidemic even among people without preexisting skin problems. Washing too often and using products have both been closely linked to a compromised skin barrier and disrupted skin microbiome. These skin care habits can cause a condition similar to genetic eczema. The lipophilic and hydrophilic properties in cleansing products strip the oil from our skin, and then they attack our stratum corneum. What finishes the job of disrupting the microbiome, breaking down the bricks and mortar, and actually leaves holes in our barrier walls? Lotions, creams, gels, serums, and masks, all of which we leave on our skin to ease the oil-stripped discomfort. They are the perfect partners in crime.

Inflammation leads to aging. Irritation leads to inflammation. What leads to this irritation? Chemicals. Where are these chemicals found?

Skincare products.

Skincare products are not the fountain of youth they promise to be. They are Father Time in disguise, stealing your skin's beauty and health!

6

EPIDEMIC

SKIN PROBLEMS AND DISEASES ARE AT ALL-TIME HIGHS

THIS IS FOR YOUR CHILD AND OLDER PARENT—NOT JUST YOUR BEAUTY

SCARE TACTICS DON'T WORK

SO FEW PEOPLE REPORTING PROBLEMS

FROM THE BEAUTY-OBSESSED SCIENTIST

THIS IS FOR YOUR CHILD AND OLDER PARENT—NOT JUST YOUR BEAUTY

Your skin is a diverse ecosystem. It is a collection of different physical matters and living, biological organisms. If this ecosystem is off-kilter, you can suffer any number of skin conditions. This book may have grabbed your attention by talking about beauty, but it is really intended to help us fight the hidden war for health.

As we have already mentioned, eczema is a prevalent skin condition affecting millions.[83] Eczema is characterized by itchy, scaly, and inflamed skin. This condition was almost nonexistent in adults prior to the 1940s and affected only about 5% of children. The '40s also marked the launch of soap operas, as you may recall. The incidence of eczema has risen steadily over the last hundred years and has skyrocketed since the 1970s.[84] Between 1977 and 2007, the prevalence of eczema tripled in the United Kingdom. Similar increases were seen in Canada, the United States, and many other developed countries. Currently, 25% of children are diagnosed with eczema. That is five times more than the '40s, and 10% of adults now suffer from this condition. Another startling correlation is that those with eczema also experience other allergic symptoms, such as asthma, hay fever, and food allergies.[85] This is the atopic march, as mentioned before, a condition in which the body's immune system reacts to things it shouldn't.

This collection of conditions is called a "march" because there is a natural *progression* of reactions triggering three pathways. The first pathway is a reaction to *contact* (the skin)—the atopic dermatitis (eczema). Dermatitis is diagnosed in babies even younger than 6 months old. Next is a reaction to substances that are *inhaled* (asthma and hay fever). This manifests in children from around 2 years of age to early school ages. The third pathway is a reaction to substances that are *ingested* (food allergies of many kinds). All of these reactions can be traced back to irritations, which are strongly linked to using products on the skin from early childhood. People who are clean- and grooming-obsessed are setting their kids up not only for skin discomfort, but also a parade of other health problems.

Both the incidence and prevalence of atopy generally are lower in developing regions of the world. The International Study of Asthma and Allergies in Childhood (ISAAC) showed that the prevalence of self-reported asthma in young teens ranged from 2% to 3% in developing countries, versus 20% to 40% in industrialized countries.[86] Why is that?

This rise of atopic disorders in the last 40 to 50 years is often explained away as a genetic predisposition.[87] It was generally believed that a person's constitution was the main factor responsible for this susceptibility. However, researchers who argued *against* this hypothesis highlighted that the sharp increase in atopy disorders happened within too short a time frame to be attributed to a genetic shift in the population. A more reasonable explanation is environmental and lifestyle changes. Cleansing and moisturizing products rework the skin's acid mantle, disturb its microbiome, and ultimately alter the skin's metabolic and barrier functions. Studies have shown that the sharp rise of autoimmune diseases in the Western world may also be caused by a disturbance in the body's microbiome in the gut and on the skin.[88] This one can't be blamed on your genetics! It is behavior-based; something you can fix if you take personal responsibility for your skin's health.

Two other papers, published in 2012 and 2014, reported that chemicals in cleansing and skincare products kick-start infants' immune systems toward atopic eczema.[89,90] The researchers made it clear they were referring to both synthetic and natural substances. Since these substances are foreign and irritating to the skin, they threaten the immune systems of developing infants. Of those children with eczema, 60% of them developed it in their first year of life, and 85% developed it during their first five years. It is clear the early years are absolutely critical in terms of how parents prepare and treat their children's bodies.

Another study, known as the "Children of the 90s Study" followed over 15,000 pregnant women and their newborns for 42 months.[91] Results showed that the "cleaner" the kids were, the higher their risk was of developing eczema and asthma. So, the more baths the kids had per week, the more likely they were to develop immune response issues. Further research has suggested a causal relationship between overcleaning and the existence of atopic diseases, concluding that sterile environments achieved through excessive cleanliness may potentially be harmful to the immune system.

Many of these allergies first manifested as sensitive skin. Sensitive skin is so prevalent that some women talk about this condition with a strange sense of something like pride, as if it means they are more precious and delicate. Plenty of medical professionals downplay sensitive skin issues as hypochondriacal whining.

Sensitive skin is not precious, nor is it trivial. It is reactive, itchy, and inflamed—a medical problem waiting to be exacerbated. It is reported that 40% of people globally have sensitive skin. Some countries have even higher rates.

A survey of US women showed that 65% of them self-reported using skincare products every day[92] (it's not clear if participants counted cleansing products as skincare). Another survey reported 69% of US women have sensitive skin. So, 65% use skincare products (likely higher), and 69% have sensitive skin! Is this a coincidence? Why is our largest organ having so much trouble?

This is not just a skin-deep, vanity issue. This is a matter of public health.

SCARE TACTICS DON'T WORK

Physicians have been warning their patients about the problems of personal care and beauty products for decades, but the approach has always come from a disease and medical perspective. That effort, I believe, is fruitless.

In her book, *Beyond Soap*, Dr. Sandy Skotnicki also addressed a series of skin problems she had seen in her more than 20 years of practice. She began with the least serious cases of sensitive skin, moved on to the more severe conditions of burning and stinging, and finally discussed the flare-ups that can come from even friction and clothing or exposure to wind and sun. This issue can be quite severe, with patients reporting feeling their skin or scalp is covered with insects, making them unable to work or sleep. The gravity of these symptoms is life-altering, and these are all real cases that parade in and out of clinics and offices every day. But *why* is talking about skin problems in this serious way *not* helpful in changing the general public's skin care behavior?

People who are obsessed with skin care usually have one goal: to make their skin more beautiful, and they believe they can only accomplish this with products. All the moderate-to-severe skin problems listed above are seen essentially as medical illnesses, but that's not what these people are concerned about.

Their primary concern is beauty. These illnesses are too serious for the beauty seekers to pay attention to. Often, the happy ending of a physician's story is, "*...and the rash improved.*" Voila, mission accomplished! Umm, no. Not to beauty-conscious women. Their mission is beautiful skin, not a disappearing rash. So the beauty seekers pay no attention to medical books or rash success stories.

"*I don't have burning or stinging skin.*"
"*My skin is not constantly itchy.*"
"*My flare-ups are pretty infrequent.*"
"*Those people must be using bad products. I choose only natural or high-end products, so I don't experience their severe problems.*"

The above thoughts are quite common in the skincare user's mind. Skincare users don't relate to clinical cases! They see these cases as people who are near the end of their rope, and their skin conditions are so worrisome that they needed a physician's help. Most skincare users are not there yet, and any talk of health and medical problems of the skin falls flat, dismissed as scare tactics.

Most people just want to know which skincare products are the best for their skin. If they can be convinced by *Skin Sobering*'s message that skincare products are *not* giving their skin beauty longevity nor are these products even good for their skin—and, instead, are harming it—then we may have a chance to awaken them from the hypnosis the beauty industry and its advertising has kept them under.

SO FEW PEOPLE REPORTING PROBLEMS

Those who seek beauty by way of products aren't primarily worried about a skin epidemic, especially teenagers and twentysomethings who are just starting to explore and enjoy products. Convincing them that products harm their skin will be a difficult but necessary first step.

Let's look at what epidemiological studies have shown us. The American FDA's first comprehensive report on adverse events related to self-care and beauty products showed the number of registered adverse events in 2013 was 291. This jumped to 436 in 2014, then 706 in 2015, and 1,591 in 2016.[93] This is across *all* of the USA! These numbers are alarming, but not just because they show a 447% increase over just three years. The real concern is that there are so *few* registered adverse events. A measly 1,500 events were reported in 2016 when 65% of women in the USA (over 100 million women) reportedly use skincare products every day, and 69% of them have sensitive skin. The disconnect here is alarming.

Now, let's examine how we think about our skin. The most common skin complaints are dryness and sensitivity. These are two symptoms that each and every one of us have experienced sometime in our product-using lives. Yet, how many of us have ever registered a formal complaint to the FDA? People view skin problems as a minor issue, and because product use is so prevalent, and adverse reactions are so frequently experienced, most people are desensitized into thinking of their damaged skin as *their skin type*, or a normal part of their skin aging or *misbehaving*. They have not realized that it is *not* their skin misbehaving. Their skin is behaving exactly as it should be when it is faced with irritants.

In other words: products.

The FDA's numbers, although small, are also alarming. Obviously, a 447% increase from 2013 to 2016, despite severe underreporting, is striking. Skin problems are not minor. Almost 80 million Americans see their doctors about their skin. In fact, skin disorders are the number one reason Americans visit their doctors, outnumbering anxiety, depression, back pain, and diabetes[94]—that's an epidemic! Even those who see their dermatologist for skin problems may not think to report those issues to the FDA or realize their condition is actually an adverse reaction to products.

Some dermatologists and academics actually question the existence of sensitive skin and claim it is merely an advertising ploy designed to sell more skincare products. They are onto something, partially. Regardless of how one thinks of sensitive skin, the conditions observed by dermatologists every day—itchiness, redness, bumps, scaliness, and irritation—are very real issues of epidemic proportions.

Returning our focus to the youth once more, the detrimental effects of overcleaning children have been so well-established that in 2016, the American Academy of Dermatology (AAD), which represents 18,000 skin-focused physicians across the world, published a "How Often Do Children Need to Bathe" guideline.[95] This stated that unless the child's skin is actually dirty, it's not necessary to bathe them more than once or twice a week. For those of us brainwashed by the post-soap opera world, this message screams "neglect," but the truth is almost the exact opposite.

Imagine how strong the evidence had to be on the *negative effects* of chemicals on the skin for these AAD members—many of whom have a mutual, interdependent relationship with the skincare industry—to make a recommendation that's bad for business. The science is so indisputable that the AAD needed to make a stand and publish what was good for people.

This recommendation from the AAD is a courageous one, no different than the Surgeon General strictly regulating tobacco and the new Canada's Food Guide deemphasizing meat and dairy. Similar to the tobacco and food industries, many dermatologists have relationships with skincare companies. Some of these physicians' main revenue sources are skincare products. The AAD's recommendation should have resulted in decreased sales for cleanser and skincare products.

At least, we hoped it would.

7

PROBLEMS

HOW DO WE HANDLE OUR SKIN WHEN WE LOVE IT AND HATE IT?

AGING. IMMUNE SYSTEM. INTERFERENCE.

SKIN-DEEP PROBLEMS AND THEIR RELATIVES

*Acne • Sensitive Skin • Dry Skin and Dehydration •
Puffy Eyes • Pigmentation • Sagging Skin*

"SKIN TYPE" EXISTS TO SELL MORE PRODUCT TYPES

END YOUR PROBLEMS

FROM THE BEAUTY-OBSESSED SCIENTIST

We all had (or still have) something we don't like about our skin. For many of us, this probably started in our teenage years, and most of us did something about it. From the first appearance of oiliness, a zit, or a blackhead, we rushed to fix it with a cleanser or a cream. We have been told that products solve problems, and there always seems to be a perfect product out there speaking to our needs.

When something minor is wrong with our bodies—a little ache, mild diarrhea, a pimple, some dryness, or a cold—we're conditioned to want to fix it right away. Of course, 9 times out of 10, that means using products. When it comes to minor complications in our body, the best way to heal and restore is to give our body time, movement, good rest, and whole foods. Our immune system is powerful enough to deal with these annoying hiccups, and it even learns how to be stronger to better combat the next problem. Of course, for serious illnesses, injuries, and broken bones, please go see your doctor!

As we get older, more problems will show up on our body. It isn't too hard to see how easy it is to blame our problems on aging. Product ads all claim to slow down aging, so why wouldn't we want those products? Aging does play a big role in us becoming weaker, especially intrinsic aging[96]—the things we were born with and can't control easily. These include our genes, race, and any inherent disease and underlying medical conditions. In contrast, extrinsic aging is due to environmental and lifestyle factors that anyone can control, if the consequences of these aging factors matter to you! The biggest extrinsic aging factors for skin are sun exposure, lifestyle choices, and the chemicals we put on our skin. These are bigger determinants of how fast or well we will age, rather than simply the number of years we've lived.

AGING. IMMUNE SYSTEM. INTERFERENCE.

When a minor issue is happening to your body, allow an appropriate amount of time to let your body do its thing before you interfere. What's an appropriate amount of time? To determine that, you will have to observe and pay attention to its progress. This is a learning process where you find out more about your own body. Monitor yourself. Is your situation getting worse (immune response kicking in) and then better (healing)? Or is your situation getting worse and worse (immune response losing and invaders taking over)? Jumping in and using a chemical right away is not giving your body an appropriate amount of time to take care of itself. When you interfere too soon, you are stealing your body's opportunity to do its job.

Examples? During childbirth, imagine the perineum being cut too quickly to widen the vaginal opening for easy access.[97] Episiotomies were standard practice in your mom's time. They were a routine procedure of childbirth which didn't allow the woman's body time to do its magic. It took the suffering of countless women speaking out against this practice before the medical and research community did something. In the 1980s, physicians finally stopped regularly cutting women from the bottom of their vagina to their rectum.

A less painful example is breastfeeding. Oftentimes, if you supplement formula to your newborn in the first few days after birth, you will disrupt the frequency of nipple suction, wreck the demand-and-supply mechanism of breastmilk production, and your milk production won't establish itself. It isn't that your body doesn't have enough milk; it is that you interfered too soon.

Another example is when you have a cold or come down with the flu. It is unwise to take antibiotics—or worse, intravenous drugs—right away. Rushing to the doctor to demand antibiotics and drugs to speed up recovery from the common cold has helped create antibiotic resistant superbugs. *Pulling the seedlings to help them grow faster* 拔苗助長 (ba miao zhu zhang) is a bang-on Chinese saying for this exact phenomenon. The seedling will look taller for a while, then eventually, it will wilt. You are essentially killing the seedling faster. Please give it time!

This principle plays out in life's other joys. My family raises 30 chickens and ducks a year for eggs and meat. When my husband and I first allowed our feather babies to roam free-range in the yard, we were concerned they wouldn't go back to their coop to roost at the end of the day. So, we frantically chased and grabbed them every evening to bring them back in. They ducked, dodged, and weaseled away as we chased them around like a pair of idiot city slickers.

After three days of this, we were exhausted and swore we'd never raise chickens again. On the fourth day, when we were hosting a dinner party and too busy to remember them, the entire flock returned to the coop—voluntarily—by dawn. My husband and I realized we had wasted a lot of time and energy chasing them. The animals would have done their natural thing all along and on their own if we'd just given them the time and the chance, instead of trying to "help" them.

With the skin-deep small stuff—a zit, blemish, oil, or dry patch—allow the natural restoring process to take place before you wash with cleansers or load up on creams that are just going to "pull the seedlings" out from under you. If you have always interfered by using products and haven't allowed your skin to do its job, your skin will be quite limited in its ability to heal and repair itself. Do not despair. If you let it, with time, your skin will break the dependent and unhealthy relationship it has developed with products. Once this happens, your skin will show you what you've wasted your time and money on, *and* it will demonstrate how you have been robbing yourself of your best skin. Allowing natural processes to happen is not neglect. Don't interrupt your body's innate work too soon by impatiently doing something to it—whether it is a puny zit or a life-giving birth.

NO PRODUCTS AND 91% OF SKIN PROBLEMS GONE

If products could make my skin more beautiful, I would have continued to use them. I did use products for over 30 years, believing that if the perfect solution was not in this one, then it would surely be found in the next. Instead, my skin got worse, despite a good lifestyle. By 53, I'd tried enough products but couldn't conceal the problems anymore. Was it just aging? Why did I keep having...

1.	large pores	12.	textured skin
2.	clogged pores	13.	roughness
3.	blackheads	14.	puffy eyes
4.	acne	15.	dark eye circles
5.	acne scars	16.	crow's feet
6.	oily T-zone	17.	dryness
7.	pigmentation	18.	dehydration
8.	blotchiness	19.	fine lines
9.	dullness	20.	itchiness
10.	uneven tone	21.	redness
11.	thin skin	22.	...and sensitivity?

I suffered from 22 annoying issues, all of which I tried to fix with products, and nothing really improved. I did look better when I had the products on, but the effect was so short-lived, like makeup. And when I was barefaced? It wasn't a pretty sight. My skin was getting noticeably worse, and the time I spent "putting my face on" and taking it off was noticeably longer. I needed two hours to get out of the house and one hour to get into bed. Thank goodness my problem list wasn't made longer by other lifestyle-related skin problems, so my time spent was still within my husband Bruce's tolerance level. Otherwise, even this famously good-tempered and patient guy would've blown up waiting for me to get out the door and deflated expecting me to get into bed.

I know I've said I quit for beauty, but maybe I should say, "For Bruce!"

After two years of *Skin Sobering*, most of my skin problems were gone. My only remaining issues are mild pigmentation and dark eye circles—conditions that take a long time to develop, so they'll take longer to resolve. Still, 20 out of 22 problems were solved. That is a whopping 91% improvement that required no money, no time, and no energy! Just a lot of determination.

That's a good score, even for Asian moms.

I have very little need to use foundation or other makeup products because my skin now looks good on its own! My overall health improved too. The money, time, and energy that I saved by dropping my "skin crack" regimen was instead spent on learning and building healthy habits. I benefited tremendously from these unexpected bonuses.

My experience is just a drop of water when it comes to the ocean of evidence Dr. Utsugi has shared from his clinical research, as well as data from numerous other scientists and their decades of studies. They conclude that products—chemicals—give you temporary visual effects and do lasting harm.

SKIN-DEEP PROBLEMS AND THEIR RELATIVES

Have you been made to believe that your skin problems are all unique and personal, as if each issue requires a different and specific skincare product? In reality, according to skin physiology and anatomy, acne, sensitivity, dryness, wrinkles, pigmentation, large pores, and many more skin issues are all close relatives. They were borne from the same ancestor and can therefore be tackled from the same root cause.

Our body is a holistic entity, and our skin is interconnected with other systems and organs, all requiring the same principle and approach to be healthy and vibrant. So we are not going to target each and every problem individually, the way skincare companies and their collaborators want you to. They sell more products that way. Let's see how *Skin Sobering* would address 99% of your skin beauty problems.

ACNE

…and Blackheads, Whiteheads, Blemishes, Oiliness, Comedone, Pustules, and More.

Let's begin with acne and its many brothers and sisters—the first skin concern to emerge during our angst-filled teenage years. At that age, even nonissues are magnified into life-altering problems, so can you imagine the typical reaction to this real skin problem? Most teenagers are bound to wash, scrub, poke, and smear.

Acne starts in the teenage years when puberty drives up hormonal activities. Hormones generate surplus sebum. This excess oil, combined with too many dead skin cells, poorly sloughed pore lining, and debris from hair follicles, results in a blocked pathway. These are the birth conditions of whiteheads and blackheads. The pathway, shared by hair follicles, oil glands, and sweat glands is the famous "pore" we are so often told must shrink and remain invisible. In this case, the pore becomes clogged. This clogging, plus the presence of the bacteria *Propionibacterium acnes* (*P. acnes*) creates the perfect environment for bacteria to grow and cause inflammation. The inflammation eventually leads to a rupturing of the oil gland, which spills its built-up contents (oil, cell debris, bacteria, and hair residue) into the surrounding tissue. The body's immune system now must respond to this erupted pore and tissue irritation with more inflammation and swelling—a necessary mechanism of healing. And voilà! You have a big, red pimple.

Armed with these anatomical and physiological facts, clever skincare companies have focused on partial science and have promoted their products according to it. They claim that their specially formulated products address the problems of acne by: (1) stripping off excess oil, (2) getting rid of dead skin, (3) killing bacteria, and (4) suppressing inflammation. It all sounds reasonable, wonderful, and even logical. This approach seems so promising, and it should make our acne go away, right?

Not really. Let's break each of them down in order.

(1) Stripping Off Excess Oil

What happens when oil is washed away from your skin? Your oil glands will secrete more to restore your skin to its natural homeostasis. When you wash with cleansers, all of which contain some form of surfactant (whether it is labeled "gentle" or "extra-strength"), you are not just washing off *excess* oil. You are stripping *all* the oil off, leaving your skin feeling pulled and dry. Some people call this "squeaky clean" as if it's a good thing! When your skin goes through repeated chemical washing, your oil glands are kept in combat mode, working to overproduce in order to fight against this constant stripping.

It is ironic to consider that in an effort to calm our oil glands—to prevent them from secreting excess oil—the skincare industry's solution in fact ended up making them overactive. Unfortunately for consumers, this results in the production of *more* acne.

And to repeat what Dr. Utsugi explained already, your oil glands eventually grow larger from this overproduction, and the pores protrude and enlarge at the same time. As the problem persists, the skin begins to resemble an orange peel. The overworked glands make the skin oily, rough, and more at risk of acne formation. Products that contain surfactants and other chemicals meant to clean off dirt and oil only add to any existing acne problem.

(2) Getting Rid of Dead Skin

How many acne products rave about containing beads meant to manually scrub off dead skin, acids formulated to chemically exfoliate dead skin, or both? It's true that science says too much dead skin clogs pores, so it appears to make perfect sense to *purposefully* get rid of these dead cells. However, as we've already explained, dead skin cells are supposed to fall off on their own.

Again, dead skin cells *need to* naturally fall off before new cells can be made. If your dead cells are not ready to fall off yet, and you *deliberately* exfoliate them, no signal will be sent. Likewise, if dead cells can't fall off when they are ready because you have goo trapping them in place, no signal will be sent either, *and* your stratum corneum thickens up from the goo. In both scenarios, your epidermis thins out from no new cell production. That's how you make your skin look ugly.

When marketing twists science and claims that you need to exfoliate to prevent dead skin buildup or acne formation, they are telling you to do *the exact opposite* of what your skin needs. Can you picture what is going on with skin that is continuously scrubbed, scraped, and drenched in products? If you imagined a thick, old, rough top layer with tons of excessive dead skin cells, you'd be right.

But wait. Isn't that the *exact* culprit for pore blockage and acne formation?

Besides the excess dead cells that are blocking your pores, the products themselves will restrict flow no matter how noncomedogenic (not clogging) they are. This is basic physics regardless of how marketing messages attempt to spin it. Think breathability. Is it easier for pores to breathe when there are chemical substances on top and inside of their small openings, or is it easier for pores to breathe when their openings are clear?

(3) Killing Bacteria

It seems to make perfect sense that if the bacteria *P. acnes* is the perpetrator of inflammation, then killing all the *P. acnes* should stop acne from forming.

Marketing and R&D professionals latch on to this argument and skillfully push their disinfecting products for acne. These products contain one form or another of alcohol, acids, melaleuca (in tea tree oil), benzoyl peroxide, or sulfur, which all have anti-inflammatory properties. However, they are also irritants to the skin and cause inflammation. This makes them a double-edged sword. How many severe acne conditions are inherent to the person's constitution, and how many are made worse by the person's own doing? I'm not attributing blame to product users here. I'm merely pointing out the widespread lack of knowledge.

Self-induced acne is not a person's fault when all they ever hear is "Use more products!"

You may have experienced this yourself or know someone with bad acne who found these disinfectants and antibiotics helped their condition. Does that mean disinfectants are effective and necessary for getting rid of acne? Many of these people are still living in an acne nightmare long after their teenage hormones have passed. Why?

Do you recall that bacteria are not just controlled by disinfectants or, to be accurate, antiseptics? They are managed much more effectively by other bacteria—the symbiotic kind. Our body has trillions of microbes. Many of them live on our skin, especially deep in our pores. We need the symbiotic ones to occupy space and produce their by-products that deter pathogens, like *P. acnes*, so they won't take up residence. A well-functioning symbiotic microbiome is our body's best and most natural means of fending off unwanted germs.

What happens when you use products with antiseptics or antibiotics on your precious face? Don't forget that these products also contain preservatives that will kill all microbes. When these preservative-filled antiseptics are applied to the face day after day, most of the symbiotic microbes are destroyed. Now pathogenic germs can take over, and *P. acnes* is one of them. People who use skincare products are unwittingly killing their good microbes and simultaneously offering a great opportunity for harmful ones to dominate and proliferate.

Instead of the intended purpose of getting rid of *P. acnes*, using these products kills your skin's army and vacates the land to allow *P. acnes* and other invasive germs to wreak havoc on your skin's health and beauty.

(4) Suppressing Inflammation

Products containing antiseptics can temporarily suppress inflammation. This is why most moderate to severe acne sufferers find these products helpful for a while. They suppress redness and blemishes, but antiseptics and preservatives are also irritants which themselves cause inflammation. Unless your skin is truly infected (not just inflamed) and needs extra help, using an antiseptic that kills *and* inflames results in prolonging your acne's life cycle and weakening your tissue's ability to heal.

During hormonal changes like puberty, menstruation, menopause, or even just day-to-day stress, you may get breakouts. In your teenage years, these breakouts can be quite bad and devastating. Let's use a figurative example to illustrate the point. Say your acne scores a 5 on a 10-point scale measuring severity, where 10 represents the worst and 1 represents the best. When you use cleansers, you think you're helping, but you are actually increasing the severity of your breakout to an 8. This is a direct result of *cleansers* drying out your skin, irritating your pores, and gearing your oil glands up to produce more oil to combat that dryness.

Your pores also get inflamed to fight the chemicals. Your Level 5 zit is now a Level 8 flare-up. You feel the urgency to treat this terrible blemish, so you use acne cream or medicated ointment to settle it down. The anti-inflammatory cream forces some surface redness to calm down, achieving a two-point reduction. It helped, you think, since the problem was brought down from an 8 to a 6.

You're so relieved, you no longer remember how it was once a mere 5.

You believe the cream is effective, and you dare not give it up. However, now you need more cleansers, even *double* cleansing to wash off the cream every morning. Yet, your skin gets drier every day. This is the classic vicious cycle where more cream needs more cleanser, which gives rise to more inflammation, which needs more cream. Just think of what these creams and cleansers are doing to your pores when you are stuck in this feedback loop.

Inflammation is the reason for your *initial* breakout and also the reason for your *ongoing* acne issues. However, there are two different sources of inflammation. The first one is bacteria-infected, which your immune system can handle. The second one is product-induced, which your immune system is not familiar with. Product irritation prolongs the acne problem.

Healing happens naturally with the help of clean water and your microbiome. With the body's normal healing mechanism, inflammation will occur as the immune system recognizes things that harm it (*P. acnes*, injuries, toxins) and sets off the body's biological defense. This manifests as mild inflammation, and it will cease a few days after harmful bacteria are successfully fended off. Your immune system wins.

However, antiseptics and preservatives are foreign substances to the body. Even though they are not exactly toxins in a chemical sense, they are unwanted by the body. These irritants drive your immune system to produce more inflammation in an attempt to fight them off. If you continue to apply chemicals, this product-induced inflammation will hang around. Then you are looking at a chronic problem.

Chronic inflammation is slow and can last for months or even years. In the case of skin health, chronic inflammation happens when these foreign irritants persist on the skin and/or when the immune response is faulty, leaving the skin in a constant state of alert. Irritation causes inflammation immediately, whether you can see it or not. Some inflammation presents itself as itchiness, dehydration, or sensitivity, which is proof that damage is taking place. Acne is a common manifestation of chronic inflammation, and the true culprit is *chemicals*—skincare products—much more so than the bacteria *P. acnes*.

Products do not help us *heal*; they help us *hide*, often ineffectively. The medicated creams pause inflammation from one source while concurrently becoming another source of inflammation on their own. Skin products go into your pores, irritate the lining, cause inflammation, and then give you more breakouts. New blemishes with redness and pus keep coming up, racing to see who can take over more skin landscape and mark more of your face. And products just prolong the outbreaks, handicapping your own metabolism.

Once you're an adult, your skin is no longer breaking out because of hormonal changes. Rather, it is doing so as a response to chemical irritations and an inability to heal. That's why my 30-year-old son, whose hormonal problems ended long ago, still has acne to deal with, plus oily skin and enlarged pores. He can't get rid of his cleansers and acne creams.

Mom knows better, son!

Acne happens during hormonal (and life) changes. So, instead of chemically stripping off oil, chemically exfoliating dead skin, chemically killing *P. acnes*, and inadvertently inflaming your skin, just clean it with water. Let it be airy and clear, and allow your skin to be sober to heal itself naturally. Acne has a short life span in the grand scheme of things, though it can be hard to convince a teenager of this. If you allow your cell renewal to function at its optimal, natural level, your acne will disappear quicker than it appeared without scarring! This undisrupted healing ability will shorten each pimple's life span. It will also help you through other hormone fluctuations to come. You'll be thankful for this knowledge when you hit menopause.

Truth Comes from Science and Data, Not Marketing

It is reported that acne is one of the most prevalent skin problems,[98] following sensitive skin. In the United States, 40 to 50 million people suffer from acne every year. In adults, the prevalence is 54% of women and 40% of men. In adolescents, the prevalence is 85%. Similar findings of 79–95% have been reported in Scotland, New Zealand, and Australia.

What does the acne picture look like in societies that do not depend on beauty products? A study looked at 1,200 residents on the remote island of Kitava, ages 10 and up. The researcher examined signs of acne and acne scarring on the residents' faces, chests, backs, and necks, and found "not a single papule, pustule, or open comedone in the entire population." Note that 25% of the population were adolescents and not one person had a pimple. Similar studies also found zero cases of acne or rates as low as 2.7%.[99]

Why is there such a startling difference between these two types of worlds? Why do almost 50% of adults and up to 95% of adolescents experience acne vulgaris in industrialized societies, versus only 2.7% and even 0% in rural societies?

Diet is the first explanation. Unprocessed foods and few simple carbohydrates mean low glycemic levels and blood insulin, hence lower rates of acne. We will discuss the importance of diet in detail in a later chapter. Another explanation is the absence of skincare products used in these societies.

Let's take a look at "baby acne" next. If you still are not convinced by acne being exacerbated by products, this is clear proof that getting rid of acne is all about healing and the repair process not being interrupted. If you've had a baby, you will remember this early skin problem. Baby acne is a result of hormonal fluctuation, just like the acne you get during puberty and menstruation. If you don't put any chemicals on the baby's skin (thank goodness even product-junkies know not to disrupt the glorious creation that is this little human), the acne heals when this hormonal spike subsides, in about 30 days. The acne doesn't come back until the next tidal wave.

You may be familiar with the argument, "Well, it's baby skin, the most regenerative and restorative skin. That is very different from older skin. Older skin needs help, so we mature people need products." Oh, I am so glad we are bringing age and restorative ability into the argument.

Let's talk about teenagers! Their bodies are young, vibrant, and healthy. Everything regenerates quickly, so teens feel invincible. They feel they can do anything and nothing will harm them. Why, then, do so many of them struggle with acne? Once it appears, it stays, gets worse, and seems to last forever!

Is it really about age? The answer is, it is about how long the teenager's hormonal fluctuation lasts and their skin's natural healing ability. And has it been disrupted or not. Teens have just as much regenerative power as babies, but by the time our babbling babies become terrible teens, most parents don't get much of a say in their daily choices anymore. By 14, most kids have indulged enough and have already "dented that perfect new car." Their exhausted parents aren't as likely to have a family meeting to discuss cleansers and creams. They have much bigger fish to fry, like sex, drugs, and bullying. By this age, kids have been exposed to a lifetime of marketing influence, so they wholeheartedly believe these products will heal their facial blemishes. So have their parents. They have long begun one disastrous skin care routine or another.

The difference between baby acne healing so quickly, teenage acne perpetuating, and mature skin showing damage is not age or regenerative abilities. It is the presence of chemicals and the mistreatment of your skin. In the case of mature skin, we've just had a *long* time to mistreat it.

Certainly, as long as your hormones are still wacky and your diet and stress levels are not ideal, you will continue to have breakouts and skin hiccups. Your best hope to have clear skin faster is not to suppress the breakouts with products. It is to give your skin the best natural chance to recover. This translates to washing your face well with just water and not putting chemicals on your skin. If you want good skin bad enough, also work on having a good diet and getting good rest and plenty of exercise.

Having a good lifestyle can be hard to achieve, but how hard is it to simply *stop putting chemicals on your skin*?

If the above is not enough to make you consider quitting skincare products, think *no scars*! Scars form when a wound is deep or when it is repeatedly inflamed and suppressed. That's exactly what chemicals do to our pores. Skin chemicals are sure to increase your chance of scarring, so break that vicious scarring cycle.

> ### TO SQUEEZE OR NOT TO SQUEEZE
>
> "I know squeezing is not good, but I want to squeeze so badly. When I see the little blackhead starting to bulge out, I know that when I give it a squeeze, the hard head and the waxy tail will slowly vomit itself out. It feels so irresistible and satisfying. I just can't hold back."
>
> You and I both know that squeezing is ever so addictive, but it's also not good for your skin. We must gauge and control our urges. If you wash your face and hands with soap and warm water first, squeeze gently with clean fingers and clipped nails and don't damage the pore (that's a skill you've got to learn first), it's okay to get the blackhead out. Knowing what is harmful and exercising some control is a more realistic goal than forcing yourself not to do it at all. A little bit of control can lead to more and better control. With *Skin Sobering*, you will find you have far fewer blemishes, and with practice, you will find yourself not needing to squeeze.

SENSITIVE SKIN
…Redness, Itchiness, Stinging, Rashes, Inflammation, Dryness, Dehydration, and More.

Sensitive skin—skin that's reactive and easily irritated—is the most prevalent skin complaint in modern societies.[100] If you have read what's written in this book so far, you can probably draw your own conclusions about what causes sensitive skin. In a nutshell, it is the accumulation of minor harm to your skin with skincare products. These harms include but are not limited to an altered acid mantle, disrupted microbiome, irritation, inflammation, and a leaky moisture barrier. All of these create a confused immune system that doesn't know how to respond anymore.

As discussed in previous chapters, a proper immune response is produced when the body senses *true* danger from an invasion. The immune system kicks into gear and triggers inflammation to attack the invaders. However, when our immune system misfires, it will cause significant inflammation and damage to our body's own healthy tissues. Hypersensitivity (allergies) and inflammatory skin disorders are the results of these autoimmune reactions.

Many of these systemic forms of allergies manifested as sensitive skin first. Sensitive skin is so prevalent that many medical professionals downplay it as hypochondriacal. As mentioned before, some women even accept it as their skin *type*. Sensitive skin is neither make-believe nor is it a skin type. It is reactive, itchy, and inflamed; it is a medical problem waiting to get worse. Sensitive skin is the beginning of many other problems.

A leaky skin barrier also leads to sensitivity. Leaky skin permits unwanted agents to get in, causing inflammation and subsequent sensitivity. How does our protective barrier *become* leaky? Leakage is the *result* of environmental and chemical attacks. When we handle our babies right from birth with cleansing and moisturizing products, we cause their skin to feel dry, and we alter its immune functioning. From birth, we begin to damage the skin.

Sensitive skin is not an innate characteristic. It is *created* through your way of living. Help stop sensitive skin by *dropping* products. Do not purchase products designed for sensitive skin. That's just marketing getting in the way of what your skin truly needs.

DRY SKIN AND DEHYDRATION

...Fine Lines, Wrinkles, Scales, Flakes, Tightness, Roughness, Itchiness, And The Seemingly Unrelated Dark Pigmentation, Dullness, Clogged Pores, Enlarged Pores, Sensitive Skin, and More.

FROM THE ANTI-AGING DOCTOR

Why are there so many people with dry and dehydrated skin? This was a puzzle to me for a long time until the answer revealed itself. No matter what products they used, the women who came to my clinic had dry, dehydrated, rough, irritated, and/or blemished skin.

The reason skin is dehydrated—the beginning cause of many problems—is because water and moisture are escaping from damaged skin. Damaged skin will also fail to protect our body from outside irritants. Skincare products assault our skin and cause it to be leaky, letting moisture get out and irritants get in. These patients were sensitive to so many things, so I suggested they try not using anything and let their skin sober up for a while.

In a month, something changed. The first thing they told me was that their skin no longer felt dry. The tight and pulling sensation they experienced after washing was gone. Their skin showed new depth and plump grains under the microscope as well.

As their skin condition improved, some of the patients relapsed and went back to their old routine, no doubt lured by the incredible promises of advertisements suggesting their products were the best and fastest way to give them instantly glowing skin. They began using skincare products again, and, as you can guess, the redness and dryness returned. This was unfortunate for the patients, but it gave me a natural, clinical, controlled trial to see the cause and effect of skincare products.

So, all these skin issues are interconnected. Dehydration, which is a lack of moisture in the intercellular channels, is caused by the compromised permeability of the skin barrier, also known as cracks in the skin.

Dehydrated skin gives rise to fine lines, crow's feet, wrinkles, and itchiness. Dryness, which is a lack of oil, can become dehydration through the use of cleansers. When oily skin becomes dehydrated, the surface corneocyte cells harden and block oil secretion. The result is that oils are trapped under the stratum corneum layer. This is a great environment for *P. acnes* to grow in.

The result? Dryness, dehydration, clogged pores, enlarged pores, and pimples! Many people don't suspect these opposing and seemingly unrelated problems—dehydrated wrinkles versus oily pimples—could be from the same root cause, but they are.

PUFFY EYES
…Crow's Feet, Dark Circles, Thin Skin, Bags Under the Eyes, and More.

There is this heated debate in the beauty world about whether one should use a specialty cream designed just for the eyes or if a high-quality face cream can do both jobs. This is the most "fun" debate created by skincare companies and their sales forces because no matter the conclusion, the consumer is convinced to use a product—an expensive "high-quality" one, for that matter. How fun is that for product sales! The debate has never been, "Is it necessary for you to use *any* product?" That's because the result of that debate might not benefit the people and corporations who produce skincare products.

FROM THE ANTI-AGING DOCTOR

Eye cream claims to improve fine lines, puffiness, and dark circles around the eyes. This skincare product is very much the same as others used for the face. So, surfactants, oils, preservatives, and additives are common ingredients. Like facial products, eye products will dissolve the intercellular substance and lower the protective barrier function of the skin. This ability alone causes the skin around the eyes to lose moisture and show fine lines and crow's feet. In addition, these surfactants and oils will lead to the same inflammation, which will result in a darker pigmentation. The inflame-then-subside-then-inflame cycle not only gives skin a darkening pigmentation, but it can also make the whites of your eyes more yellow. If you pull and rub the skin around the eyes, these negative effects magnify.

When you apply eye cream, it gives the skin's surface a temporary illusion of moisture that lasts until the product is dry or comes off. During this time, fine lines seem less visible. The more eye cream you use, the less likely the skin will be able to exfoliate naturally, reducing signal send-down, halting new cell division, and slowing metabolic activity. The result is a thinning of the eye epidermis—the same negative effects that face cream has on the rest of your face.

The thinning of this already thin area has a worse aesthetic effect. The vessels and muscles under that skin become much more visible, making the eye area dark and veiny. This occurrence is best known as dark under-eye circles. These three attacks—moisture barrier loss, inflammation, and thinning of the skin—are the result of using eye cream (or luxe face cream). They are a contributor to eye beauty problems, not a cure.

So, does the skin around our eyes really require products? Why isn't there any eye product research comparing no cream to any cream? Every advertisement compares one product against another and claims their product is superior, be it more eco-friendly, luxurious, effective, or whatever they want to say. "One jar of Olay cream hydrates better than five jars of the prestige cream." All products make enticing claims, but most have led to disappointment. If this isn't the case, then why are we always looking for the next product and falling out of love with the ones we bought and believed in before?

A note about genetics: if you've had bags under your eyes since you were a kid, then you have more fat there than you'd like. This is what you were born with. No cream, serum, lotion, or *Skin Sobering* is going to do anything for that, nor is there any clinical treatment involving lasers, peels, or injections that will make a difference. Only surgical removal of the fat will work, and that is a risky option with plenty of reasons to avoid it.

If your puffiness appeared later in life, it could be from allergies, lack of sleep, or more likely, products. Try eliminating products first before you turn to surgery!

PIGMENTATION
...Blotchiness, Dull Skin, Dark Spots, and More—Plus Pigheadedness.

Hyperpigmentation is *my* beauty Achilles heel, and it is widely misunderstood. Most people only know the two most common culprits: UV rays and hormones, and aren't familiar with the other two big perpetrators: inflammation and thin skin.

I don't have beautiful skin according to Chinese standards, or more accurately, the whole Asian world. First, my skin is not fair. We have a saying in Chinese 一白遮三醜 (yi bai zhe san chou) *one white covers three uglies*. It means fair skin is so beautiful that its presence is powerful enough to hide three ugly facial features. Culturally, being fair or white is *that* important to Asians. Second, my pores are visible. I have good, strong pores that pump out a lot of sweat, and we know sweat glands and pores go hand in hand. Many of my people have porcelain skin and no pores visible to the naked eye. They were born that way. Third, I have freckles and other dark spots. My mom has even more because her generation didn't know about UV protection. Even though I am very careful with the sun, my inherent pigmentation characteristics are here to stay.

To Asians, pigments are flaws. We don't think Annie or Pippy Longstocking are pretty. My friends called me "map face" but since I am thick-skinned, I survived the teasing. I didn't, however, overcome the self-doubt. My "three uglies" combined with my Amazon woman's height make me unattractive to the Chinese world. 林黛玉 (Lin Dai Yu), a sickly principal character in the infamous Chinese novel *Dream of the Red Chamber* 紅樓夢, was considered extremely beautiful—one of the most beautiful women in Chinese literature. Beauty was fragility! To some extent, it still is. Korean makeup techniques emphasize a soft, delicate, and shy appearance, like using reddish eyeshadow to make it look like you just cried. So vulnerable! 楚楚可憐 (chu chu ke lian)—*adorable and pitiful!*

That's not me.

The reality is that genetics is king when it comes to skin beauty. Even though my skin has improved remarkably since *Skin Sobering*, I was born, according to Asian beauty standards, with just B-quality skin, at best a B+. A person may see me and think, "Your skin is not that nice. So-and-so has way prettier skin than you, so I'd rather listen to what she has to say." It's a struggle to get people to follow someone's advice when she doesn't have Instagram-perfect skin, despite how much it may have improved from its condition before.

When you are in search of self-improvement, avoid comparing yourself with others. Instead, compare against yourself. When you are looking for sound advice, listen to those who've made the biggest improvements, not those who were born gorgeous. Genetically gifted people had much less to do with their enviable characteristics than Instagram and advertising would have us believe. When I compare my skin today to 3 or even 10 years ago, I have only 2 of the 22 problem conditions I used to struggle with. My skin has gotten so much better and healthier that I only need to spend 10 minutes instead of 2 hours on my face before I go out the door. My friends may not notice a big change because they were only allowed to see the most *naturally made-up face I was willing to show them*. I showed them a face that took me two hours to create each day. I know what I looked like when I scrubbed and cleansed everything off. Now, I proudly show people the 10-minute, clean, and natural me.

When I decided to write this book, I knew my skin would be judged. Please do not judge me on my genetics. I had nothing to do with that. Judge me on my improvements. That's my doing.

Hyperpigmentation is exacerbated by UV rays, which we all know. However, I avoid the sun like the plague (except the first summer when I arrived in Canada), so that's not the main cause of my pigmentation issues. Melasma and blotchiness are triggered by hormonal changes, a problem of mine as I gave birth to three healthy boys in five years. But I treated my "map face" with laser technology, which helped to remove surface sunspots. So my hyperpigmentation wasn't due to either of the two most common reasons. It was a lesser known (or, at that time, unknown) reason: chronic inflammation caused by skincare products. Ingredients like surfactants and oils made my pores red and inflamed. This mild inflammation persisted because I kept using products. Of course, the products prolonged the inflammation and induced dullness and pigment production. My skin turned patchy and lost its glow.

Chronic inflammation played a leading role, but there was another supporting star at play: thinning skin. As you may remember, when the dead corneocyte cells get sticky and cannot naturally exfoliate, no signal is sent down to make new cells. The epidermis eventually thins out, and the vessels, follicles, and muscles in the dermis can show through this translucent layer. The result is pigmented blotches.

Products that were marketed to give me younger and more beautiful skin didn't work. Not using products and practicing *Skin Sobering* returned my skin to its best state. Today, my skin is supple, smooth, and clear, with normal oil production and visually smaller pores because of no more clogging. When all of that happened, it dawned on me that I didn't mind the color of my skin so much. When my skin was dull, plugged, and dry, I hated my freckles and yellow skin. But it was actually the dullness and the gray tone I was fighting against, not my innate skin color and characteristics.

If you're born with oilier skin, that's your skin. If you're born with yellow skin, that's your color. If you inherited bigger pores from your dad instead of my best friend Lan's porcelain skin, that's your complexion. You can't change your inherent characteristics and definitely not from the outside (unless you go under the knife).

Unfortunately though, you *can* damage your skin from the outside. When obsessing over your skin with a fine-toothed comb, know what you were blessed with (things that can't be changed) and what you have altered (things that can be changed back). If you fail to recognize this difference, you are bound to spend a lifetime, tons of money, and massive amounts of energy fighting against your natural skin, ultimately making it worse. My fighting cost me decades of wasted time and money, and my skin ended up worse for it.

My lovely stepdaughter and future daughters-in-law are wiser and kinder. They convinced me that I have beautiful skin according to Western beauty standards. First, my color is great, like a mild tan. The warm, yellow coloring the Asians dislike, the Caucasians appreciate. Second, I don't have any wrinkles. At 57, I don't have many fine lines, although I had a lot around my eyes prior to *Skin Sobering*. Third, my skin is firm and not sagging. I credit this to my diligent use of physical sun shields (I wear a full sun mask to cycle even in 30 degrees Celsius weather) and to living a healthy lifestyle. Finally, these lovely ladies even supplied me with a fourth factor to appreciate: my freckles make me look cute and younger. Thank goodness I'm living here, and thank God for such great daughters.

So, this section is not so much about pigmentation but rather the pigheadedness that can come from one's personal hang-ups. We could spend our whole lives trying to correct a problem that others often don't notice, or that they may even think is your strength. I still don't have porcelain skin, but since my pores are no longer clogged, they are much smaller. And I don't have ugly, unhealthy skin anymore either.

SAGGING SKIN
...Jowl, Poor Elasticity, Deep Wrinkles, Withered Skin, and More.

There are some skin problems that even *Skin Sobering* cannot change. For these conditions, remember that if *Skin Sobering* can't help—that is, your skin's own regenerative power—products have no hope of helping either. These conditions include collagen loss, sagginess, train-track wrinkles, RBF jowls, leathery skin, and problems directly related to genetics, sun exposure, diet, and lifestyle.

No matter how many skincare products you use or how diligently you practice *Skin Sobering*, none of these listed issues are salvageable. However, even though products can't improve deeper layer functioning, with daily, long-term use, they *can worsen it*. So, whether you do or don't suffer from major skin issues, *Skin Sobering* is still the best way to care for your skin.

If skin products won't work and *Skin Sobering* can't fix the issue, what's one to do? Don't worry, there are lots of little devices on late-night commercials and specialty beauty stores that promise to fix all our problems. An experienced plastic surgeon, Andrew Jacono, wrote in his book[101] and warned readers that any device advertised to tighten your face, neck, or other skin—like a roller, or a massager with some radiofrequency, sonic, or electrical waveform—is not going to work. The reason why facial tissue sags is because it has been stretched out by gravity, rubbing, and tugging for many years. The jowl forms not because your face or neck muscles are *weak* but because they've *changed shape*. So, no matter how much you exercise or stimulate your face or neck, those muscles are not going to retract.

Some will say that advocating *Skin Sobering* reveals a hidden agenda behind plastic surgery. It may. Their hidden agenda, if there is one, is to bring you to *their* independent business. However, the decision not to invest in "miracle" creams and devices does not necessarily translate into deciding to undergo plastic surgery. Plus, the decision to get plastic surgery is not going to translate to you going to their specific clinic. There are lots of plastic surgeons to choose from. If there's any conspiracy here, it would only work if there were huge conglomerates promoting a one-sided, system-wide message where they control such a substantial portion of the market that no matter what you buy or where you buy it from, they win.

Um, who has that kind of power? That sounds so familiar.

If your mind jumped to the beauty and skincare industry, you'd be right.

INVASIVE PROCEDURES

To truly "reverse aging," you'll need much more radical interventions. Fillers, Botox, or plastic surgery all come with risks, and the risks are often greater than the problems themselves. We are *not* advocating plastic surgery or any invasive treatments. We are mentioning them to make it clear that *no* skincare products can remedy "aging" conditions or truly fix other minor ones. If you do choose to go through with invasive procedures, be aware that the risk is high and rates of dissatisfaction are even higher. You mostly see successful cases, usually just through photos, and this is known as "survivorship bias." We see this concept play out in restaurant businesses all the time: over 90% of new restaurants fail, but we don't see that. We see only the ones left standing, which can make it seem like opening a restaurant is a great business idea.

What's the failure rate in invasive cosmetic procedures? First of all, it's too hard to define "failure" for something subjective like attractiveness. Does it have to be a botch to be a fail? What if the client didn't get exactly what they expected out of the procedure? And what's the incentive for treatment providers to report or even collect accurate data when the conflict of interest is so high? It's best for this industry that we know nothing about disgruntled clients and just ignorantly come get ourselves fixed.

Remember, the beauty industry is so loosely regulated that there's no governing body to enforce data collection or reporting.

I've been thinking about plastic surgeries for myself, like getting my nasal labial folds flattened, but I cannot bear to take the risk. Plastic surgery is an "all or nothing" deal to me. If the result is not *exactly* what I want, I will be permanently altered.

No one plans to go through plastic surgery to get just *sort of* what they want. If I'm going to spend all that money, have my face cut open, and endure the pain, I'm not going to be happy with just an "okay" result.

You want exactly what you want, and that is hard when you start to alter nature. You may indeed find the very best surgeon who listens, understands, and has the artistic and technical skills to perfectly translate your hopes through their knives, but in reality that is a rare stroke of luck. The chances of cosmetic and surgical procedures not working exactly how patients envision them are high. Look at all the celebrity no-so-rights and unnaturalness! Can you think of a celebrity whose face looks "wrong" after they've undergone plastic surgery? These people

> have all the money and resources to find the best surgeons with the best skills. They can travel anywhere in the world to receive the best and most artistic care, and still so many of their results look less than enviable.
>
> Instead of altering nature, we would be wise to make every attempt to preserve and heal what we already have. We can start by eliminating the use of skincare products. That's the easiest route.

"SKIN TYPE" EXISTS TO SELL MORE PRODUCT TYPES

Skin-typing is a brilliant way to sell more products. With a uniquely formulated product for each "type" of skin and for each part of our body, skincare companies can cater to our every desire and insecurity while raking in the cash. They try to tell us we are special people with unique needs who deserve *something* (make that *many things*) formulated just for us. They make sure you know your skin could be dry, dehydrated, oily, a combination, sensitive, or (God forbid) normal. Then, they fine-tune even more to arrive at the "perfect" product for you. You will need something completely different if you are a baby, a child, a teen, an adult, over 40, over 60, female, male, trans…The list goes on. Even if we didn't think we needed products, this carefully customized approach is designed to make us feel distinct from ordinary people so we'll want and buy special products.

This marketing strategy is even more cunning than horizontal segmentation. With horizontal segmentation, companies change the smell, color, and package of the products. Here, they try to change us.

Are we really born with so many natural differences? Do those differences really require so many different products? Do babies have different skin types? They do, but with a much narrower range. Some babies are a little oilier, some sweatier, and some have more melanin, but that's about it. Despite what beauty and skincare companies try to make us believe, when we are born, our skin is pretty similar. As hormones kick in during adolescence, all people's skin will change somewhat, primarily becoming more—more oily, more sweaty, more smelly. But as powerful as hormones are, external factors, such as the sun, harsh elements, the stuff we consume, the lifestyle habits we pick up, and the products we put on our skin affect its characteristics much more. It is managing these factors, especially the easy one—skincare products—that will make the biggest difference for your skin.

So, skin types aren't really highlighted for the purpose of skin health. No one worries about skin types for babies, and they shouldn't. The idea of skin types was manufactured to sell skin products. We have been conditioned to focus on the minute differences of our skin, rather than its holistic health.

I saw a brilliant marketing scheme on a Canadian talk show called *The Social* in late November 2020. This one will surely make you buy multiple products. It's called *multi-masking*. The beauty expert said you need one mask for the tip of your nose, one for the groove of your nose, one for your T-zone, one for your forehead, one for your cheeks, one for under your eyes, one for your crow's feet, one for your laugh lines, one for your chin, one for your neck...

Wait, how many masks have I mentioned so far?

Instead of buying one mask (which is already one too many), you're now spending 10 times the amount of money, 10 times the amount of energy, and doing 10 times the amount of harm. What a brilliant, bullshit idea. And the women on this talk show were oohing and ahhing over their Picasso-like, masked faces, believing they were getting firsthand access to the latest revolutionary beauty technique. If the TV station is making advertising money by endorsing these products, okay fine. They are a business, and this is a common business practice. But if the hosts actually believe in multi-masking? Let's just say, I would love the opportunity to share this science with them and help them *truly* make their skin healthier and more beautiful.

Always check the science. Please don't let marketing blind your reasoning.

My stepdaughter just wrote me as I was editing, "Oh, random thought, did you know there are beauty creams for your butt now?"

Excuse me, *what?*

Oh, this makes me mad. First there was just cream. Then there was cream for the face and hands; then came creams for the eyes, lips, neck, decolletage, body, and feet. Now there's cream for your butt? Seriously? The butt *is* part of your damn body! You don't need a different cream for your butt. You don't need a cream for *anywhere* on your body! This industry is trying so hard to bait us to spend, spend, spend. Who cares if your skin suffers, suffers, *suffers*?

The multi-masking and 10-step gimmicks are obviously too extreme for some. "I do things in moderation, and I strike a balanced approach," one might rightfully proclaim. This flattering Goldilocks notion of using the "just right" amount of products is understandable. For most of us, our understanding of skin care was influenced long before we knew how to reason and think critically.

When it comes to skin care and skincare products, let's think of *moderation* the way we do when we think about smoking cigarettes. When it comes to lighting up and ingesting carcinogens, *even a little is too much*. The moderation sentiment doesn't work well here.

If you *know* skincare chemicals are *bad* for you, and you choose to use them anyway—even in excess—that is your right. But I'd bet my bottom dollar that those who talk about moderation in this case actually are unaware that skincare products are just like tobacco, alcohol, and sugar. My passionate preaching doesn't mean your life can't include any unhealthy choices. You deserve to *know* the true effects of the things you use—the good and the bad, and then you do you. Fair game. But if you've only heard information from people who are positioned to profit from you, then that's not fair. You are not making an informed choice.

Keep in mind that doctors, our most authoritative health figures, are now the world's second-largest sales force for cosmetic and skincare products![102]

"Our skin is all different, so we need different products to care for it." That's another load of crap, once again created by marketing. Consider listening to someone claim, "Our lungs are all different, so we each need different things for them," or "Our livers are all different, so we need different things for them." This claim of extreme individuality is just a sales tactic devised to push a wider variety of skincare products. We are more similar than we are different, and the needs of our organs are quite universal. Our lungs need fresh air and exercise. Our livers need less fat and less alcohol. Our skin is an organ that needs good rest, exercise, clean water, and protection from the elements.

We're of the same human type; we are not all that different.

END YOUR PROBLEMS

Mistreating the skin leads to lots of problems. We can end each of them by choosing not to mistreat our skin anymore. We know sun exposure and sugar damage the skin. Is using skin products a mistreatment as well? If you have read the previous chapters, you know this is a rhetorical question. If your skin feels dry, end that by eliminating the use of cleansers and don't apply any moisturizers. They serve only to mask issues and break down your moisture barrier. If you feel oily, end that also by eliminating cleansers as they strip the natural oils off your face. They will only make your glands produce more oil. If you have acne, end that by throwing your lotions and potions in the trash. They will only clog your pores and inflame them further. If you have sensitive skin, end that—you guessed it—the same way.

Skin is the most misunderstood and mistreated organ. We are hooked on the skin care industry's temporary fixes like the drugs they are. They provide us a great look while eroding our skin layers we can't immediately see. The damage is nowhere near as severe as "moon face or shrunken balls" from steroid use; we get that. After all, it's just skin. But the *disparity* in terms of how much you believe in the goodness of skin chemicals compared to how unaware you are of their hidden damages is the seriousness of this. When it comes to other drugs, at least we know they are for short-term use. We already acknowledge they will cause damage if we use them inappropriately and long-term. By contrast, we have been taught to think of skincare products like nutrients, and we indulge in them too freely and too frequently. That's the worrisome part.

Stop using skincare products. That's how you can begin to end your problems.

8

GUIDE

HOW TO BE SIMPLY BEAUTIFUL WITH SKIN SOBERING

UTSUGI'S METHOD
Cleaning—Your "Gateway Drug" • *Skin CARE ≠ Skin Chemicals* •
Makeup—Yes, You Can • *Microscopic Examination—To Tell the Truth*

SO MUCH CLEANSING

GIVE YOUR SKIN A CHANCE TO HEAL ITSELF
Cold Turkey vs. Fasting

APRÈS-SKIN SOBERING

FROM THE BEAUTY-OBSESSED SCIENTIST

Skin Sobering isn't about *not* using makeup. It isn't about sacrificing looks, and it certainly is not about neglecting your skin. *Skin Sobering* is about giving your skin its best chance to be beautiful and healthy. The best way to achieve that happens to be eliminating the use of skincare products and breaking your skin's dependency on them. *Skin Sobering* for this beauty-obsessed scientist is about having the best natural canvas to put makeup on when I want to show my glammed-up face.

Skin Sobering won't stop you from getting old. I have practiced *Skin Sobering* since 2019, and I don't look like a 20-year-old. But I think I'm a fine-looking 57-year-old, with my proud living marks. I have gone through the stress of giving birth and raising children, the pressure of making it in my careers, the tension of relationships, the heartbreak of caring for the old, and the worries of life. Oh, and the effects of sunshine! I won't stop playing outside. Those things are unavoidable for me and have added up to give me age signs everywhere, especially on my face. Those were not problems for me.

The problems I detested were the *accelerated* signs of aging that were in fact *avoidable*. The fine lines, pigmentation, large pores, clogged pores, dark eye circles, puffiness, blemishes, acne scars, sensitivity, oiliness, dullness, dryness, thin skin, thick skin, rough skin, ugly skin—all these "beauty by-product" problems that were chemically produced and should *not* happen to a 57-year-old face. Thankfully, after *Skin Sobering*, those unappealing issues have almost entirely healed and vanished.

Skin that has been affected by chemicals (whether the product claims to be natural or synthetic, as well as cleansers—by this point in the book, I realize this is your millionth reminder) has lost some degree of its innate metabolism. The degree of this loss depends on how frequently, how much, and how long a person has used skin chemicals. Once skin is functioning normally after *Skin Sobering*, you can use skincare products to brighten up your look in the same way you'd use makeup. But please realize that this "brightening" comes with a cost: the cost of cumulative damage.

You may need more than a book to get through this journey, just like with most other habit changes. But if you understand the science and have the persistence to allow your skin to complete its withdrawal and regenerating process, you won't need supplementary help. The book itself will be enough. Many people can quit drinking and smoking, or successfully adopt a healthy diet and exercise routine on their own after they have digested knowledge that empowers them to make the change. It is the same for *Skin Sobering*.

FROM THE ANTI-AGING DOCTOR

UTSUGI'S METHOD

It is shortsighted and sad to only chase today's brief beauty, to look good now and ignore what will happen later. Be careful with the allure of instant gratification, and render your skin not aging well. You can still prioritize today's beauty if you are equipped with knowledge of skin and skincare products, and if you know how to adjust according to your skin's changes. Our skin has incredible regenerative capabilities, so the good news is that even if you have been altering and harming your skin for decades, as long as you stop damaging it, your skin will bounce back. People who practice Utsugi's Method for skin care the *Skin Sobering* way in their 30s, 50s, or even their 80s are all proof of this.

To care for your skin, the most important thing is to keep its natural innate functions working well and for as long as possible. *Skin Sobering* is simple, and it is your skin's best chance to achieve optimal barrier functioning and skin metabolism. It takes time and consistency for our bodies to change in a lasting way, but practice and persist, and you will restore your most beautiful skin.

CLEANING—YOUR "GATEWAY DRUG"

Most of us began the vicious cycle of product use with a cleansing "drug." We start much earlier than we realize, as teenagers or even as babies, and we pump up the volume when we see signs we don't like. When you don't accept that it is normal to have increased oil production and acne during puberty—which, if properly handled, should be of reduced life span and severity—and rush in with chemicals, you help start an unfortunate and harmful cycle. We strip our skin of its natural oils, which causes it to produce more oil or dryness, and makes it abnormal. Then you soothe your skin with more products, which irritates it and induces blemishes, more oil, and more dryness. All these products were supposed to help you. Instead, they help each other and leave your skin craving another hit. At that point, you can't stay away from any products because they all appear to be so necessary.

According to a 2022 skin care market report,[103] the two bestselling products in the US are facial cleansers and acne treatments, pushing 304 million and 85 million units respectively in 2020. Great business, poor skin!

So, the first step you can take to help is to stop washing with these gateway products, namely cleansers. While cleansing products effectively strip all the dirt off your skin, they also take away your innate moisturizing and protective substances and predispose your skin to dryness, irritation, and deeper problems. Pick a day to begin a new cycle of not putting anything on your skin, and try washing your face with water alone. Don't let your previous beliefs take over your sense of reason. You don't need any of those products; your old beliefs are just fueled by the most glamorous "drug industry" on the planet.

Warm water is powerful. It can sufficiently clean sweat, dust, sebum, mucus, urine, and blood off of our skin. You don't need anything else.

Some may complain, "I can't let the flaws on my face show." Those flaws are exactly the skin problems that skincare and makeup products exacerbate or even create. Let's not continue that feedback loop. If you can make it through your skin's withdrawal phase, you won't need the coverage much longer.

The purpose of cleaning your face is to wash away the day's dust, dirt, and most importantly, lipid (squalene) peroxides. Oils secreted by our oil (sebaceous) glands oxidize within a few hours when exposed to air and free radicals. These lipid peroxides are not good for our cell membranes, so they must be washed away. Even though these peroxides are oils, the ones oxidized from your own sebum and sweat with no skincare products added are water-soluble and can be effectively washed away with lukewarm water.

Pollutants in the air also won't stick to your skin much if you have not layered it with products. This is the double jeopardy of skincare products: they harm your skin on their own, *and* they attract more pollutants to stick to your skin. These cause further harm, yet the clever lie skincare companies have been telling is that skincare products *protect* us from pollutants. This is nonsensical—just think of physics and particle adhesion.

What is lukewarm water? Our body temperature is about 36 to 37 degrees Celsius. On the skin's surface, that temperature is about 1 to 2 degrees lower, around 34 to 35 degrees. Your wrist is a good testing tool. So if the water doesn't feel hot or cold on your wrist, it is the appropriate temperature to wash away most oils, odor-causing sulfides, oxides, and dirt. Being hygienic doesn't mean being so "squeaky clean" that your skin is tight and pulled. Don't let years of advertising and misconceptions beat your sense of reason.

Do not increase water temperature in colder seasons. You may find the heat feels good in the moment, but the higher the temperature, the more it will dry your skin. In the morning, it's best to use cooler water. There's not much oxidized oil or dirt on the skin at this time, since you likely just cleaned it the night before, and if you don't sweat heavily at night. Cleaning off eye sand and washing your face gently with cool water will not only be good for your skin, but it will also rejuvenate you.

Wash with Your Hands

Your hands are the best tool you have for washing. There's no need to use a sponge, cloth, or brush—and please, avoid motorized rotating brushes! That's how floors are cleaned, not faces.

Here is how to clean and preserve your face. Cup your hands together and fill them with lukewarm water. Place your face in the water and lightly press your palms to your face. This likely isn't how you've washed your face before, as it involves no rubbing or scrubbing. Move the cupped water around the various sections of your face in an orderly fashion. Start with the nose, eyes, and mouth, and then move across to your cheeks, temples, and ears. Next, move up to your forehead, then down to your mouth and chin. Repeat this cupping motion a few times with clean water, and hold the water against each section of your face for a few seconds so it can soak into the dirt a bit. This will enhance water's effectiveness. Think of dirty dishes: when you soak them, the dirt comes off so much easier. The pressing motion will gently pulsate the water between your palms and face, further dissolving the dirt.

With clean water in your hands, *glide* your palms and fingertips across all sections of your face. Use your palms for your cheeks, chin, and forehead; use your fingers for your eyes, nose, and ears. This gliding motion is not to be confused with rubbing, which you should not do. If, while washing your face, you notice your skin moving with your hands, you are applying too much pressure.

This method seems so basic, yet most people have washed their face the wrong way. Washing in this manner is to ensure the water is cleaning and buffering between your hands and your face. The stratum corneum is only 0.01mm thin, and it is even thinner around your eyes, so the goal is to be gentle. If the corneum is rubbed off prematurely, your skin will flake more and age faster. After washing, use a soft, clean cloth to dab your skin dry. Remember, just dab. A soft cloth is a good drying tool, but not a washing tool. New cloths usually have oil in their fibers, so they are not very absorbent. Wash them a few times before using them on your face. Because the skin doesn't like water residue to be left on it, people tend to rub their skin dry. They are often unaware of the excessive force they are applying. Do not rub or scrub.

If you like to shower, you may use the showerhead to rinse your face, but the temperature must be just below your body temperature and the pressure must be low. If you enjoy a high-pressure spray, that will disrupt your natural moisturizing barriers and cause your skin to feel dry. Use the high pressure and heat on your back and legs where the skin is not as delicate. It is best to shield your face with your hands and let the water indirectly wash your face.

How to Use Soap

Note: If you've ever heard that soap is the worst for the face, you may wonder why we are giving it credit here. Please read along to get other scientists' reports—those who are unattached to the beauty industry, like us.

There's no need to overclean. If you don't smear substances on your face, even pure soap is unnecessary, and its use should be limited. Cleaning with *any* products is the gateway to dryness! Stop that first, and you won't need to smear products on your face to ease that dryness. Powder makeup can be cleaned with warm water alone. Your hands, however, should be frequently cleaned with pure soap and water. Poor hardworking hands.

When you must put foreign substances on your face, then you should use soap to clean them. The key benefits of using pure soap to clean your skin are its gentleness, as there are no synthetic surfactants. Use suds, as they can dissolve oil and dirt by bringing them to the surface of the skin. Suds can also act as a lubricant, so your hands won't be rubbing your skin, and your stratum corneum won't be hurt. Lather up some rich suds to the size of a ping-pong ball, and wash your face using your palms and fingers. Put the suds in your palms and press them against the skin. This will make the bubbles collapse. Then, slightly release the pressure and allow the suds to create a little suction between your hands and your skin. The suds will naturally work their way into your skin's grooves to gently and effectively pull up dirt. Repeat this a few times without any rubbing or pulling. You should apply even less pressure when you're washing near your eyes, like you are touching tofu. Remember again that the stratum corneum is only 0.01mm thin, so treat it more tenderly than tofu.

When you are done, rinse all the soap suds off of your face using the cupping method. Ensure you have fresh water in your cupped hands each time, and then bury your face in the water. This gives the soap a chance to dissolve in the water. Move your hands along your face in the same manner as described before. Don't splash, don't miss any spots, and repeat this 10 times. The main thing to remember is, again, not to rub, scrub, or pull the skin. Just apply gentle pressure with your palms and fingers.

And there's no need to use even pure soap on your face if it's just your own secretions and airborne dirt on it. Pure soap will also dry your skin. So less chemicals the better to care for your skin.

SKIN CARE ≠ SKIN CHEMICALS

We have heard our moms (and even grandmas) say we must moisturize, moisturize, moisturize. We have been convinced it is the most important aspect of skin care. What we should actually be focused on is *moisture, moisture, moisture.*

Skin care is all about *keeping moisture in* and protecting our skin against external and internal assaults—not *moisturizing* it. The skin care method that is best for health and beauty is one that keeps our *own* moisture in and everything else out.

If you have exposed your skin to chemicals and the damages of the world and your skin is already dry, how do you bring your moisture back and reverse that condition? It is certainly not by "moisturizing" and using chemicals applied from the outside, as we have been led to believe. In earlier chapters, we learned that the first and foremost reason our skin is dry is because we clean it with chemicals—face wash, cleansing lotions, cleansing creams, makeup removers, oils, and toners. The surfactants in these liquids are powerful oil strippers. Cleansing with chemicals is what started the skin's drying state in the first place. Moisturizers also contain plenty of surfactants and other damaging substances. They exacerbate this dryness while they sit on the skin. All the time they spend there allows them to break down the skin's natural barriers further. When the skin is subjected to daily cleansing and moisturizing, it becomes leaky in no time.

Test this. After you clean your face, leave it bare. If it feels dry or tight at all, your moisture barrier is compromised by products. "Helping" your skin by slathering moisturizer from outside is just masking the dryness temporarily, while deepening the compromise. Moisture is leaking from *within*. *This* is transepidermal water loss (TEWL).

No amount of moisture applied from the outside will prevent the leaking of internal water. So the only way to help the skin retain its own moisture is to stop its protective barrier from being broken down any further. By now, you know exactly what your skin needs—no cleansers or leave-on products.

Retaining Moisture of Disrupted Skin

When your skin is dehydrated or dry, the edges of the stratum corneum cells will curl up, like BBQing squid, causing the skin to peel prematurely. If the source of that dryness (chemicals) isn't stopped, cracks will form. These tiny cracks and lesions that allow the transepidermal water to leak are not visible to the naked eye but can certainly be felt. Dryness is the most common reason for itchy skin. As you have likely learned by now, this is a sign of inflammation. Moisture loss and mild inflammation are the root causes of many other skin problems.

When the skin is already dry, dehydrated, or leaky, the only way to immediately help it to retain its own moisture and prevent further TEWL is to add a moisture *barrier*, not a *moisturizer*. As mentioned in earlier chapters, pure petroleum jelly, commonly known by its name brand "Vaseline," is most useful at this point because, despite being a chemical, it is inert and 100% pure. Vaseline will smooth the curled-up edges of the stratum corneum and hold them in place to prevent further moisture evaporation. Vaseline can also shield the skin from outside irritation and allow the lesions to heal, provided the chemical attacks don't continue.

When you first stop using skin chemicals, or when humidity levels are low, your skin may feel dry or flaky. To ease this feeling, a small amount of Vaseline is helpful. After you truly sober up your skin, your moisture barrier will gradually regenerate itself and prevent moisture leakage. Dryness will diminish, and you won't even need Vaseline. Give it time, and one day you will suddenly notice your skin feeling soft, supple, and looking good. By then, you will not feel the need to help your skin with Vaseline and definitely not with skincare products. A clear and smooth face is very attractive and a wonderful base for some occasional enhancement.

If you are wondering whether or not you need Vaseline on a particular day, a key guide is if your skin *feels* itchy or dry. If it doesn't, there's no need to use Vaseline or anything else. Not applying anything topically is the fastest way to get your skin to its optimal condition, though there are some exceptions. If the relative humidity is below 30%, or if it is a dry winter, you can use a very thin layer of Vaseline around your eyes and on your cheeks to ease weather-related dryness. If your lips are dry, or you have a habit of licking them (which will only make them dryer), you may apply some Vaseline there as well. Vaseline acts as a *barrier* against the elements and against your saliva. Other forms of lip products—especially medicated lip treatments—that claim to "moisturize" your lips will actually dry them out faster than you realize. In fact, the more products you put on your lips, the drier they will feel. Your lips are extremely sensitive, so they will show the effects of these products the quickest.

Some people find Vaseline sticky. That's just a matter of the amount used. Don't use too much—that's most people's mistake. When you see disastrous videos on YouTube of children's hair covered with Vaseline, that's because these kiddies scooped out half the jar! If you use Vaseline sparingly, that sticky sensation will disappear after a few minutes. The way to avoid overusing Vaseline is to spread a dot the size of half a grain of rice on your wrist with your fingertip to warm it up. Don't apply it directly onto your face by rubbing it on. Once the small dot is thinned and warmed, dab a thin film of it onto your dry areas. For the larger parts of your face, warm a larger dot in your palms using a circular motion, then press it onto your cheeks or forehead. Always use a clean cotton Q-Tip to scoop the Vaseline out of the jar. This will help keep the bacteria count low.

Recall that Vaseline's inert nature means it won't oxidize, so it won't cause any harm to your skin while it's on there. Vaseline also doesn't need to be washed away with soap. Water alone will suffice. The small amount of Vaseline that remains after washing can help protect your skin the next morning, so there's no need to reapply it. Don't forget: stripping your skin clean is worse for it.

But also remember, you shouldn't overuse anything—not even Vaseline. It will dry your skin out as well. Imagine using plastic wrap to cover your skin. Within minutes, the water and moisture in your skin that wants to evaporate would be trapped under the plastic wrap. A thick layer of Vaseline behaves the same way. When moisture can't naturally air off, it will be reabsorbed by the stratum corneum cells. This will affect natural exfoliation. The eventual evaporation of water in the cells will not only take moisture away, but it will also remove your natural moisturizing factor, making your skin dryer and weaker.

Once your skin's health has been restored, the dryness will go away. At this point, you no longer need anything on it. When your skin doesn't *feel* dry—no pulling, itching, or stinging after you wash it—don't even use Vaseline. Occasional flaky skin is normal. That's your skin exfoliating naturally, so don't mistake that for dryness and reach for moisturizers again. When you stop using *chemicals* to *clean* and *care*, your skin's own moisturizing factors will take charge and do their job. If you have to face the world and are bothered by the small flakes, dab on a bit of Vaseline before you apply makeup.

After your skin health is restored, as long as your rate of chemical use is less frequent than your skin's renewal rate, there will be very little harm done when you use makeup to beautify.

WE DON'T SELL VASELINE®

Vaseline has gotten such a bad rap. It's hard to make people understand why this 100% petroleum jelly is your skin's second-best moisture barrier without going into chemistry and skin physiology.

Petroleum jelly (PJ) is a petroleum-based by-product of mineral oils and waxes. Vaseline®, a proprietary brand of PJ, has gone through a triple purification process of distillation, de-aeration, and filtration, making it the most inert, pure, and least irritating substance out there.[104] Because PJ is nonperishable, there are no preservatives in it either. PJ's property also won't change for years, unlike plant oil or animal fat, which will oxidize once exposed to the air. In the early days, PJ was used in rhinoplasty and breast enlargement because of its stability. But a few years of stability is not long enough for the purposes of an implant, so that was stopped. Vaseline also won't be absorbed into the skin. Not being easily oxidized nor absorbed means that PJ will not trigger any irritation, so used in moderation, it is a harmless product for our skin.

Why use an inert substance that doesn't go into the skin, instead of a moisturizer that penetrates? The simple, physiological answer is that hydrated skin comes from within. We can't help our skin to be hydrated topically by trying to moisturize it from the outside. We can only prevent transepidermal water loss (TEWL) from within. A thin film of Vaseline will sit on top of your skin and won't get into your pores, so your sweat can still secrete. Don't be alarmed by the fact that it's petroleum. It's so purified and "natural" that physicians use it for skin ulcerations, burns, and treating traumatized skin to protect the lesions.

Disclaimer: Neither Dr. Utsugi nor Dr. Tjam have any affiliation or financial connection with Vaseline or its parent company, Unilever. They are simply speaking about chemistry and physiology. The Vaseline brand now offers many lotions and creams that are NOT 100% petroleum jelly. These new Vaseline-brand products possess the same harmful elements as other skincare products. We do not recommend them.

UV Protection

UV rays from the sun give plants life and give us happiness. Unfortunately, they are also a big skin beauty offender, causing photoaging and many other skin health problems. The ultimate way to avoid the damage of UV rays is to avoid exposing your *face* to the sun. Let your legs and arms do the sunny job of getting Vitamin D and other goodness. You should play outside, and you should use physical shields as much as possible to protect your face. By "as much as possible," I mean shield up until it is too bizarre of a look for the culture you live in.

There are a lot of new sun protective fabrics on the market that can block over 90% of UV rays, like hats with wide rims, ball caps, face masks, and umbrellas. Walk in the shade and under awnings whenever possible.

When it is not possible to use a shield, or when using it looks worse than skin damage itself (This makes Dr. Tjam think of the plastic cover her aunt kept over her sofa!), using sunscreen products is the lesser of the two evils.

Most sunscreen products come in the form of a lotion or cream, so they also dissolve our NMF, destroy its protective barrier, and cause the skin to be dry. In addition, removing sunscreen will involve using cleansers and rubbing, which further accelerates the breakdown of the barrier. All of these combined could be more harmful to the skin than a small amount of UV exposure itself—even I, an Asian who is vehemently against sun darkening, am okay with this.

Many sunscreen "educators" are urging people to wear sunscreen even indoors and under LED lighting. Being so fearful of UV rays that you end up wearing sunscreen 16/7 (accounting for eight hours of sleep) will make the lesser evil a much more prominent one. If you are exposed to the sun for less than 20 minutes a day, just wear a hat. That's much more effective for UV protection and skin health.

MAKEUP—YES, YOU CAN

During the withdrawal period when your skin is recovering and not looking its best yet, or when you have some special VIP to see, it is understandable that you may want to brighten your look. Some key area makeup is good; just be aware of what you are doing.

Key Area Makeup

If your only concern is to have healthy skin, of course then it's best not to apply makeup at all. However, using makeup in many societies is considered good etiquette. It gives people more confidence and is pleasing to others around them. So, there may be times when you want to elevate your look and don't mind sacrificing your skin a bit. In these circumstances, please use key area makeup. Key areas refer to brows, eyes, cheeks, and lips. Under the microscope, one can see that makeup in a few areas is a lot less damaging than applying it on the whole face, especially when it comes to liquid foundation.

Use pure mineral, loose powder makeup when you need to enhance your look. Loose powder doesn't contain oil or surfactants, so it's much less damaging to your skin than liquid or cream makeup. The powder offers a natural coverage and an illuminating effect. Powders come in brilliant colors and can be found in the form of foundation, eyeshadow, brow colors, and blush. If you think powder foundation looks dry, give your skin 15 minutes to let the powder settle with your own natural moisture before you go out. The longer you skin sober, the more efficiently your own moisture will return and the dewier your makeup will look.

Do not use concealer, primer, or tinted moisturizer prior to the loose powder foundation. These products have the same harmful ingredients as liquid and cream skincare products. The more you use, the worse your skin will become. If you have spots or blemishes that you must cover, use a bit thicker layer of pure mineral powder mixed with water. You may also seriously ask why these flaws are there in the first place. Are skincare products contributing to their presence, and do you want to exacerbate these problems? Helping your skin to regain its renewal ability and heal scars and blemishes is the true solution—and sober skin can do just that!

Beauty-conscious people likely won't want to give up their makeup entirely for the sake of healthy skin, so key area makeup is a good alternative. Your skin will recover from its damaged and flawed state slightly slower if you choose to use makeup, but you may find this to be a more acceptable way of balancing skin health and beauty during the intermediary recovery phase.

Don't forget that unhealthy skin is the reason most women feel the need to use large amounts of makeup in the first place. Even with key area makeup, please don't use it every day. You must have days where you can tolerate being barefaced. The more of those days you can experience, the faster your skin will restore. If your skin is itchy, dry, flaky, or covered in blemishes, give it a rest for at least three days. Don't *sprinkle salt on the wound* 傷口撒鹽 (shang kou sa yan) and add insult to injury. Use nothing until these problems subside.

Use Vaseline as a Primer

When loose powder foundation feels dry because your skin hasn't gained back its natural moisturizing factor yet, you may use Vaseline as a primer before applying the powder. Vaseline is an excellent choice because, if your skin is damaged, there will be very little grainy network in your skin. That's why the powder won't stay. Before your skin recovers and regains its healthy texture, Vaseline can be used to help your makeup stay on smoothly. Again, your own oil can smooth out powder foundation too, so allow some time after washing your face before you apply powder foundation.

If you need to attend an event and want more covered-looking skin, you may have to use a concealer or liquid foundation. In this case, dab a thin layer of Vaseline first to create a barrier between your skin and the harmful makeup. This will reduce the harm done by the makeup; though, again, it is not an ideal situation for your skin.

Eyes. When applying mineral powder eyeshadow, it's best to use a soft brush and dab it on gently, not brushing back and forth. Cream or stick shadows have to be rubbed on, which induces more stretching. For eyeliner, the worst type is pencil form. Pencils are much harder, so you need to use more pressure to apply. In order to have a precise line, many people will tug the outer edge of their lids to smooth out the skin. Over time their super thin stratum corneum and delicate muscles will loosen, causing them to sag and pigment (the "droopy eyelids" or "triangular eyes" syndrome). I've also heard that blending is important for color mixing, but there's a trade-off between skin tautness and blended colors. So, please don't overdo it.

A lot of my patients have itchy and stingy eyes. When I examined them under the microscope, I saw the skin around their eyes was inflamed with dark, accumulated residue. This is eyeliner-related contact dermatitis causing inflammation, dryness, and itchiness. Skin that is chronically inflamed will become hyperpigmented, and when this occurs around the eyelids, they become dull and loose. The same science you've learned about skin applies to your eyelids as well.

Applying liquid foundation or concealer on your eyelids is a big no-no. You may want to do this to cover up dark or dull eyelids, but this will only add to your initial problems, making your lids darker and duller. The actions in removing this foundation also harms your eyelids.

To prevent these foreign substances from sitting directly on your eyelids, lightly dab on a little bit of Vaseline before any eye makeup. This can reduce the harm caused by eyeshadow and liner. Again, there's no need to stress about thoroughly removing the Vaseline. It will fall off during your natural skin exfoliation cycle within a few days.

Mascara is very popular, and all my staff use it. They ask, "Dr. Utsugi, I am not putting it directly on my skin, so why does it matter if I use mascara?" Is it really harmless if the product is just on your lashes? I studied the eyelid skin of mascara users under the microscope and discovered that the skin around the lashes was all red. This redness was not detectable by the naked eye. If this inflammation persists, the eyelids will darken. Further, if the inflammation doesn't subside, the whites of the eyes will also become inflamed. Collagen inside the whites will build up, and the blood vessels will enlarge. These will cause the whites to become dull and muddy, and your eyes will dry as a result.

It is not an exaggeration when we say *Skin Sobering* will even brighten the whites of your eyes!

Lips. Lipsticks, gloss, and balms have become essential for many women. No matter which kind you choose, they all contain surfactants. The more types you put on, the more harm you are doing to your lips. That's why almost everyone I know has dry lips. If you want to minimize the harm, just use one type, and remember that the thicker you apply the product, the more surfactants you're putting on your lips. So, please go thin.

Lips are formed with a mucous membrane and have a natural reddish sheen when they are healthy. When you attempt to acquire this reddish sheen using lipstick, it penetrates your skin and causes inflammation and pigment precipitation. You end up damaging the membrane, dulling your lips, and defeating the entire purpose of the product. So, use them wisely with this knowledge.

How to Clean Off Makeup

When you are removing mineral makeup, do not use any liquid cleansers (particularly not makeup remover). Just use water, or a little bit of pure soap suds. There's no need to overclean. The powder makeup mentioned above can be washed off effectively with water alone. However, if you need to use liquid or viscous makeup occasionally, you will need to use pure soap to wash it off. Otherwise, even pure soap is unnecessary, and its use should be limited.

If you apply makeup to your eye areas, you'll need to pay special attention when washing your face. Use your fingertip to glide over the area gently, and do not rub. If you cannot remove the makeup using just water, add some pure soap suds. There are some mascaras that are water-soluble, which are less harmful for your eyes. If you want water-resistant mascara, choose one that will come off like silicone particles when you finger-brush along the lashes. If you can refrain from using liquid foundation, you won't even need to use soap and will eventually have no *need* for any foundation.

Lipstick only needs to be wiped off with facial tissue. There's no need to do anything further. When you apply lipstick the next day, yesterday's minute residue will blend with the new lipstick. The skin on our lips regenerates very quickly, so any residue will fall off in two or three days. If you use soap or other removers to pull lipstick out of the lines and folds of your lips, you are forcefully removing your NMF as well. This will leave your lips dryer and coarser.

It is not necessary to strip your face completely clean of infrequently applied makeup, contrary to product-driven, popular belief. Even some doctors feel this way, especially the ones "trained" by cosmetic companies. The more important message that doctors should deliver is to allow your skin many periods of chemical-free rest. If there's a bit of makeup left on your skin, the surface skin will flake off, so that makeup residue will fall alongside it anyway. It is much more damaging to take off your skin's natural protections than to have a bit of makeup remain.

As we continue to pursue beauty and perfection—demanding immediate effects—we actually end up with persistent dullness, discomfort, dryness, and even decreased vision. Is it worth it? Don't apply makeup every day, even if it is key area makeup. Only use it when there is a worthwhile event that deserves the damaging of your skin. Hopefully, you don't have these events every day. Healthy, bare, and natural skin (a.k.a. sober skin) reflects energy and vitality. That is real beauty.

When you are young, the above advice will seem pointless. Most of your damages will recover on their own. But you won't age well if you continue this behavior.

MICROSCOPIC EXAMINATION—
TO TELL THE TRUTH

An effective way to thoroughly examine our skin's beauty and health is to use a digital microscope that can be connected to a computer monitor. A handheld microscope with a magnifying power of 30 to 500 times (50 times being the most applicable for the skin) can display the skin's condition clearly. Skin texture is magnified to show the surface grains, pores, and epidermal pigmentations, as well as to reflect the vessels and collagen fibers in the dermal layers. Trained eyes can also use the microscope to detect dullness and inflammation.

The skin condition of my "product-addicted" patients seemed fine to the naked eye, especially while the products were on their skin and their condition had become chronic. When we examined their skin using the microscope, the good grainy texture was so hard to detect. It was shallow and undefined. Not only that, but their pores were also red and inflamed. The skin around their pores had darkened from this inflammation, resulting in hyperpigmentation. Since these blemishes were just around their pores, not all over their skin, it was hard for people to notice the damaging effects of products. This chronic invisible inflammation can escape the naked eye, but not the microscope.

A microscopic examination is very important for clinical assessment. This kind of handheld microscope can also be used by anyone to see the true condition of their skin. It is a helpful tool to observe your skin through the

> stages, to establish a baseline, and to monitor your progress as your skin improves.

FROM THE BEAUTY-OBSESSED SCIENTIST
SO MUCH CLEANSING

If your skin feels dry, first take a look at how you clean it. When it comes to dirtiness, first look at what you put on your skin. As a matter of fact, when it comes to sensitivity, itchiness, oiliness, and dehydration, they all relate to how you clean your skin. When it comes to dullness, fine lines, puffiness, pigmentation, large pores, dark under-eye circles, they all have something to do with what you put on your skin.

Dermatologist Dr. Skotnicki used the terms "clean-obsessed" and "product-junkie society" to describe how we as a nation misunderstand our bodies. We wash, buff, exfoliate, moisturize, slather, hydrate, and soften endlessly, fearing that we are not clean enough. In turn, we interfere with our skin so much that we force it away from its healthiest condition. We've forgotten what a wonderful creation the human body is. We appear to have globally forgotten the remarkable abilities of our largest organ and how it can naturally moisturize and protect itself. So, the most important thing you can do for your face is to *not* overwash it, especially with products.

Unless your job involves getting a lot of external substances on your skin—perhaps you work in an oil refinery, cook over a greasy wok all day, or you *have to* cover your face in cream and makeup—water alone *can* efficiently clean off body secretions and airborne pollutants. Your face does not hold onto handrails or touch toilet seats, so it is not exposed to the same dirt and germs as your hands. But when you choose to *put* dirt on your face—natural or synthetic oils, colors, fragrances, preservatives, and surfactants (a.k.a. makeup and skincare products)—you then have to use chemical cleansers to clean them off. What irony!

If you still are not convinced by *Skin Sobering*, or your lifestyle simply won't let you stop putting products on your face, start with your body, from the neck down. Just use water on your *body*, and let that part of your skin show you how good *Skin Sobering* is.

WHAT IS PURE SOAP?

Soap has a bad rap, just like Vaseline.[105] Here, we mean bar soap, or more accurately, pure soap. Pure soap only comes in bar form. There are other bar soaps that are not pure soap, so it is important to understand what pure soap is in order to ensure we're buying the right thing.

When it comes to using bar soap, many immediately think of touching someone else's wet bar and getting their germs. A study found that even with deliberately contaminated bars of soap, the bacteria on them wasn't transferred during hand washing. This is because soap and water trap germs and dirt in the suds they produce, which makes bar soap essentially self-cleaning. The ick factor is just imagined.[106]

Soapmaking is called saponification, a chemical reaction where fatty acids and an alkali react to produce soap and glycerol.[107] The alkali is usually lye, and the fatty acids can come from animal fats or plant oils. Today's soaps have gone through many rounds of purifications, making pure soap milder and lower in PH despite its alkaline nature. Soap molecules have one end that bonds with water (hydrophilic) and another that bonds with oils and fats (lipophilic), so it is a natural surfactant.[108] When you lather up suds, the molecules effectively lift dirt, oil, and germs away from your skin. Then, a rinse with water washes everything away.

What is *pure* soap? Beauty advertising has long used the terms like *pure* and *natural* to appeal to nature-minded consumers, but it doesn't mean their soap is pure chemically. When we say "pure soap," "basic soap," "true soap," or just "soap," we mean a soap that consists only of fatty acids and alkali without any extra ingredients. If a soap has more than five ingredients, it's likely not pure soap. So, check the ingredients label. Many of these extra ingredients are impurities in the form of alcohol, sugar, wax, paraffin, silicates, and flour that function as fillers and binders. Others add milk, fruits, flowers, and many bizarre mixtures into soap to imply some imagined, enhanced, and "natural" benefit. These ingredients cannot be put on the skin without heavy chemical extraction, ironically making most infused soaps entirely unnatural. Soap's job is to clean, not to moisturize, so the simpler the soap, the gentler it is on your skin. As with the skincare products we've already debunked, conditioners added to these fancy soaps may leave you with a temporarily "moisturized" feeling, but really? The sensation simply comes from chemicals left behind to break down your skin. That impure soap will irritate your skin more and cost you more.

Not all bar soaps are pure. Soap can come as a syndet bar or a combar, and both contain many synthetic substances. *Syndet* means synthetic detergent (yes, it is a detergent, like the one you use to strip grease off your dishes), which is a term for surfactants that are made synthetically.[109] It is present in all liquid and many bar forms. Clinique, Dove, Oil of Olay, Vel, and most beauty soaps are syndets. *Combar* means combination bar, which is soap and syndet combined. Because syndets and combars both have high levels of skin moisturizers, they leave the skin feeling soft right after use. However, the surfactants and additives in the moisturizers also break down your skin barrier and leave your skin dryer when the moisturizers are gone.

Pure soap is more alkaline than syndets and combars, and this characteristic has been used by beauty professionals to label soap as "harsh" and something that will disrupt your skin's acid mantle. But our skin has an impressive buffering capacity,[110] which will neutralize the mild alkalinity and restore the skin surface back to its acidic state in less than half an hour. The purity and simplicity of pure soap leaves no trace of chemicals, unlike the high quantity of surfactants and moisturizers found in syndets and combars. They are much more harmful to the skin than soap, despite providing a short-lived feeling of softness.

It is worthwhile to point out that the carbon footprint for liquid cleansers is 25% more than bar soap. Consumers also use seven times more liquid soap than bar soap. So, pure soap is better for your skin and for the environment—and you also pay less for it.

GIVE YOUR SKIN A CHANCE TO HEAL ITSELF

Another irony is that skin without products will renew faster and heal better. That translates to an aesthetic and physical end result of better-looking and healthier skin. Life has a lot of hiccups, as does this excretory organ—a little bump, a bit oily, a tad dry, a slight itch, and more. These are normal conditions, and your body will heal them. Don't reach for chemical help right away.

It is normal to be a bit abnormal!

Clean unsightly areas with lukewarm water a couple more times if there's a bump or oiliness; use cooler water if it feels dry or itchy. Then wait. Give your skin time to get through the condition. It will, and it will get through it even faster the next time if you refrain from interfering with products this time. Conversely, if you always lather up or smear on the moment you see a blemish, you are taking away your skin's own healing ability. Eventually, skin treated this way will have a hard time healing completely. Once that happens, your skin will look sick—that is, chronic oily, dry, sensitive, itchy, dull, clogged, puffy, and so on. That skin is not beautiful, and now it is abnormal as well.

If you don't feel there's anything wrong with the products you use because your skin is not suffering from any of the symptoms we've discussed, then your ability to heal is winning over product damage. But remember two things: One, our body's healing power will weaken in time, so be careful of the product damage sneaking up on you while you are blissfully oblivious. Two, why are you using products in the first place if there isn't *anything* wrong with your skin? You've been blessed by genetics, but if you continue to challenge your genetics by using products that you never even needed in the first place, your skin will age and worsen faster and faster. You won't age as well as you could be.

Practicing *Skin Sobering* doesn't mean you will have no skin problems. Your skin is a living and constantly regenerating organ, so depending on the ebbs and flows of your body, you will see normal problems. For example, skin naturally exfoliates, so your skin will flake off periodically. Our body sheds about 40,000 (or 12 grams) of dead skin cells per day. This equals about 4 kilograms a year.[111] Most people can't lose that much weight in a year. Dead skin flaking is one of the most normal bodily functions.

DOS AND DON'TS

Suppressing your skin issues is easy when using drugs and chemicals. However, that doesn't strengthen your regenerating; instead, it weakens that ability. There are a few common skin issues that will keep appearing simply because our internal and external environments keep changing. When these problems occur, don't jump to products. Give your skin time to go through its normal cycle. Here are some dos and don'ts to help you work through the hiccups.

Blemishes

Whether it is acne, redness, oiliness, or sensitivity...

Do:

- Wash your face with lukewarm water at night and in the morning, and dab dry.
- Limit your intake of dairy, sugar, and simple carbs, especially when you have flare-ups.

Don't:

- Apply any chemicals to suppress the blemish, even anti-inflammatory compounds. They will irritate your pores further, making it harder for your immune system to complete the healing cycle.

- Wash with any cleansers, toners, or acne products. Skin without products is easy to clean. Sweat and sebum can be washed off with lukewarm water.
- Use any concealer or cover-up. This one is hard, because we usually don't want anyone to see our blemishes. If you must use a cover-up, use it only when you are seeing people (loose mineral powder has good coverage). Wash it off with warm water immediately after you get home, and let your skin rest.

Flaking

When products are off your skin and no sticky goo is on your skin, you will see flakes every few days. That's your skin doing its work properly. The flakes will be much smaller as your skin gets healthier, and there will be no dry feeling despite some flaky looks. Skin that's no longer damaged will have nearly invisible flakes, like baby's skin.

Do:

- Wash with *cooler*-temperature water to reduce drying.
- Sweat through exercising. Exercise is great for your skin, and fresh sweat is your skin's natural moisturizer.
- Let sweat stay on your skin for an hour or so. Fresh sweat is not dirt.
- Wash off your sweat with cool water after a couple of hours, as oils do oxidize.
- Dab a very thin layer of Vaseline to smooth the flakes if you need to face the world and cannot tolerate any tiny flakes.

Don't:

- Put on any lotion or cream to conceal the flakes. This is another temporary fix that will worsen the problem and make

it last longer. Your skin will be gooey and won't be able to exfoliate and regenerate naturally.
- Ever exfoliate manually or chemically. That will exacerbate your flaking problem as you are forcing skin cells to come off before they are ready. That's injuring your skin, like peeling off a scab.
- Wash with any "moisturizing" products or wash more often. You need to give your skin time to get through the flaking.

Dryness

When you *feel* pulling, tightness, or itchiness, your skin is dry or dehydrated. *Seeing* flakes doesn't mean your skin is dry.

Do:

- All the same Dos in "Flaking," plus...
- Dab a very thin layer of Vaseline as a moisture barrier to reduce TEWL. Spot treat dry patches instead of applying Vaseline to the whole face.

Don't:

- All the same Don'ts in "Flaking," plus...
- Wash with anything other than water. All products will further weaken your moisture barrier, making you drier.

To put it simply, all skin beauty issues are best healed by *Skin Sobering*.

To take it up a notch, *P*rotect from the elements (P), and *A*djust your lifestyle (A). Together, with *Skin Sobering* (SS), your skin and health will be in its top form. The concept of PASS will be explained in more detail later.

FASTING (THE FOOD VERSION)

If you still don't know that fasting is one of the best things to step up your health game, please read or listen to Jason Fung, Peter Attia, David Sinclair, Valter Longo, Rich Roll, James Clear, Tom Bilyeu, Tim Ferriss, and the least well-known one (with almost no followers on social media), Yoshinori Ohsumi. He happens to have won the Nobel Prize in Medicine in 2016.

I'm deliberately not including celebrities in this list, only people who have studied fasting, written about it, or been invited by the scientific community to speak about it, to give this lifestyle practice credibility. All these people have discovered fasting and have made it part of their life of pursuing health and longevity.

COLD TURKEY VS. FASTING

When you first try *Skin Sobering*, you can do it one of two ways. You can go cold turkey, especially if you are staying at home or wearing a mask most of the time. Not having to show your face during this adjustment stage helps. Or you can do it gradually, like fasting (as it relates to food). This is not to imply that chemicals are nutrients like food, so "skin fasting" is not the same as traditional fasting. They just share a similar process, name, and hurdles.

If you have eaten three meals a day (plus snacks!) all your life, to quit a meal or not eat for any length of time is going to make you *hangry*—hungry + angry! You will miss food, want food, and want to kill for food. The same goes for quitting skincare products. We apply our products first thing in the morning and usually don't take them off until we're ready to go to bed at night. Then we put the night creams right back on. These products stay on your skin literally 24/7, far longer than food stays in your stomach. So, just like learning to fast by slowly cutting back on the number of times you eat each day, *Skin Sobering* can be approached in the same gradual and gentle way.

When you decide to start food fasting, it is recommended that you drink lots of water and just hold off eating for as long as you can. You may not make it past breakfast the first time you try, and that's okay. Note how you feel and how long you held off, then let yourself have food. The next day try again, note how you feel, and try to last a little longer than you did the day before. After a few days of trial and error, you will have learned how your body reacts and therefore how you can ride each hunger wave as it arrives (which is truly a wave, because your hunger hormones will subside and your feelings of hunger will fade). The next day, you'll find you can last longer. Eventually, you'll be able to completely skip breakfast. (Note: Breakfast is not the most important meal of the day. Breakfast brands have done a fantastic job "educating" us to never skip their sugary goodness.) Great! Stick to no breakfast for a month, then try to get past lunch. Once you are able to go 24 hours without eating, your body has adjusted to fasting. You can now more safely and successfully participate in longer fasts and set your length and frequency according to your health and goals.

Starting *Skin Sobering* gradually can be a good option for many. If you can't sober up your skin for more than a day because you are feeling so dry, greasy, or itchy (that's your skin manifesting its damages and acting up due to withdrawal), then use a bit of product to help it adjust. First, start with Vaseline to see if it helps to soothe the dryness and itchiness. Alternatively, use more water to take away the greasiness. If you just can't get used to Vaseline or water, then go back to your old product but begin cutting back from there. Skincare products are not as toxic as drugs, so you can reduce the amount to 1/2, 1/7, 1/30, by only using them every other day, every week, and eventually every month. If so, hey, you are doing *Skin Sobering*! Every time you reduce, you're giving your skin much-needed recuperation time.

Think of *Skin Sobering* like healthy eating. You may set a goal to eat healthy every day, but it's hard at first. So, by the fifth day you cave, and you shove chips down your throat. Don't beat yourself up. Know that healthy eating, like exercise, is a cumulative and lifelong process. Maybe you caved today. So what? Don't think, "The hell with it!" and completely fall off the wagon. Get back on the horse tomorrow because you know this is good for your health. Hopefully this time you will eat healthy for 10 days in a row. Hopefully this time, you can go even longer without products.

When you restart the *Skin Sobering* clock, allow yourself to monitor, adapt, and extend the sobering time. Just like food fasting, now you know how your skin reacts when there's no products on it. Now you know what it feels like to fight through the waves of withdrawal. Every day you don't use chemicals, your skin gains much-needed rest and renewal. It is good to restart and to go longer each time. Not many people can *reach the sky in one step*—步登天 (yi bu deng tian) or "build Rome in one day," so quitting your products gradually is okay.

The worst part about building a good habit is that we all have the initial momentum to get started, but excitement dims as the boredom of repetition emerges. This usually happens before people can see any encouraging results, and it isn't uncommon for doubt to slink its way in. One of the worst attitudes to have is "all or nothing," like, "I can't do this perfectly, so I'm not going to do it at all." All-or-nothing thoughts are the enemy of building any good habits. If you can't be perfect, that's okay. Just be *something*. Self-loathing serves little purpose, but persistence will lead to consistency. As Jane Fonda so famously said, "Don't try to be perfect. It's a losing battle, and you'll just be unhappy.

Your anxiety will drive you to do things like eat too much or drink too much or whatever."[112]

It took me three months to get my skin sober. I was able to quit skincare and beauty products cold turkey. I worked through the withdrawal phase without caving in to products. When you know that not having chemicals on your skin is good for your skin, just like when you know eating vegetables is good for your health, it is much easier to keep at it. That's what worked for me, but it's okay if cold turkey doesn't work for you. You don't need to follow any particular path—just do it your own way. Truly, any method you choose to achieve sober skin is healthier than continuing a lifetime of damaging product use.

Some may argue that a single weekend without makeup is surely enough rest for our skin, and that there's no need to quit entirely. Think about cigarettes and drugs. If you quit smoking for a single weekend, have you truly detoxed? You need to completely stop smoking for an extended period of time to be sober (or in this case, smoke-free). However, after you've gained full control of your habit, when your body (skin) has regained its metabolic functioning, you *can* use products sparingly. Unlike with truly addictive substances, after you've succeeded in fully kicking the skincare product habit, you'll find you're able to function like a nonaddict. You can even enjoy the occasional "puff" (or serum) without going right back to the habit. My husband smokes a good cigar on special occasions, and there's really no harm done. He's in control. The same principles apply to skincare products.

Many people actually forget or dread their skincare routine because it *is* such a pain in the neck. COVID-19 changed our face-the-world routine, so most people stopped fussing over skin care and skipped the enhancement. Many looked haggard (it was because of wearing sweats, a messy bun, and no haircuts) despite developing better, healthier skin. The sad thing was, without the knowledge of *Skin*

Sobering, most people *thought* that they were neglecting their skin and got right back to "caring" for it with products as restrictions began to lift. When I told my friends the principle of *Skin Sobering*, they happily replied, "Great! I don't have to feel bad about *not* doing the usual skin care now that I know it's good for me!" We hope this book will give you the confidence that comes with knowing that the responsible thing to do is to quit the chemicals.

APRÈS-SKIN SOBERING

After *Skin Sobering*, the very first thing you will notice is that your skin will heal a lot faster, and it will heal *completely*. Your regenerative abilities will bounce back to what they were when you were younger. That means if you get acne, it will heal quickly. If you have a rash, a dry patch, or any of the other things that your skin goes through because you are a living being, those issues will heal faster and more thoroughly too—that is also the best beautifying process you can dream of.

As I've already shared, I still use skincare products for those rare, special occasions when I really want to glam up. Now that my skin has revived, I need very few chemicals to feel confident with my looks. My skin base is good, so there's not much for me to conceal. I even dare to pull my hair back into a messy bun in public now. I feel wonderful that I am not putting any chemicals on my skin, and I am satisfied knowing this is the best for my skin.

When I'm deciding whether to use skincare or makeup, I ask myself if this function is important enough for me to damage my skin. If it's my wedding, I'm going all out for the day. I'm moisturizing, masking, using serums—anything to make me look temporarily unnaturally gorgeous. It's my day! When I'm attending my best friend's wedding? Oh, yeah! I'm not just damaging my skin that day, I'm torturing it a few weeks before with heat, chemicals, and needles, then creams and lotions, just so I can look not even like myself, but like a star. That comes from a true story and, sure enough, my poor skin suffered. The damage showed up shortly after my best friend's big day and stayed for a long time. Thank goodness my friends and I have not been married that many times, and thank goodness for my après-*Skin Sobering* skin that is healthy and regenerative. I no longer need to constantly torture my skin for my friends' big day. As my Bruce often tells me, I look naturally gorgeous (that's just blind love talking).

Thank goodness for Dr. Utsugi, who showed me that *Skin Sobering* is the best way for my skin to renew and beautify itself. So, even though I cause some damage once in a while, I know damn well to stay away from products for at least twice as long as I would put them on my skin. Most of the time when I go to an event, I just need powder foundation and key area makeup. For my usual outings, I put nothing on my skin, opting instead for a stylish outfit (even my ski, cycling, yoga, and pickleball gear are on point, I must say). I am feeling more confident with no products on my face, because each day, my skin looks better and better. Hearing about it or reading about it is one thing, but experiencing the power of sober skin is the most convincing data one can have. The more time I give to *Skin Sobering*, the better I am *aging*.

SUCCESSFUL SKIN SOBERER

There are umpteen ways to achieve different health habits. In diet alone we have Atkins, Zone, keto, vegetarian, vegan, Weight Watchers, South Beach, raw food, Mediterranean, Western...and proponents of each rave about their way being the best, most efficient, and simplest. When it comes to skin care, of course we believe *Skin Sobering* is the mother of all methods. A Toronto-based dermatologist previously referenced in this book, Dr. Skotnicki, has commented on living with sober skin, evidently benefiting more from *Skin Sobering* than her own method.

Dr. Skotnicki gave a lot of great advice in her *Beyond Soap* book. Her own experience gave a lot of great proof for the value of our *Skin Sobering* way:

> In 2014, I joined an expedition to the North Magnetic Pole, to raise awareness of Canadian military veterans. Nights required enduring temperatures that sank to 25 below zero. I was one of the many members who'd never done anything like it. When I told my friends, they had questions. "How on earth will you wash yourself?" What a reflection on our obsession with cleanliness that washing would come up so early in any discussion.
>
> We were on the Arctic ice for eight days. Each night I'd wipe myself down with a paper towel and a little warm water. I went without a shower for more than a week. We made it to the North Pole and back—and I didn't smell. But here's what really blew me away. When I stepped into my hotel, I was afraid to look in the mirror. But what I saw surprised me so much that I still think about it years later. I peered at my reflection for the first time in a week and discovered that my skin was *glowing*. For more than a week, all I'd done was use sunscreen and rinse my skin off once a day with warmed artic snow. My skin was the best I'd ever seen it.

If Dr. Skotnicki thinks back to this experience she had eight years ago, the only thing she did was wash her face with warm water, and that took off even the greasy sunscreen she was using. She didn't use any of the soaps, syndet, combars, or liquid cleansers that she analyzed in such detail in her book. She didn't need moisturizer, even when facing harsh Arctic weather daily.

How long did it take before her skin was glowing?

Eight. Days.

Without realizing it, Dr. Skotnicki practiced *Skin Sobering* for merely eight days and felt her skin was the best she'd ever seen it! *Skin Sobering* works, not just for skin illnesses but surely for skin beauty too.

And in her own words, "rather than using more products, whether organic or synthetic, what could be more natural than leaving the skin of the body to care for itself?" We could not agree more with that conclusion!

9

PRODUCTS
...AND PROMISES WITH NO PROOF

PHYSIOLOGY FOR PRODUCTS

COMPANIES' CLAIMS ARE TO GET YOU TO BUY

*Product Safety • Dermatologist Tested • Fragrance-Free •
Preservative-Free • Hypoallergenic • Cosmeceutical • Subjective Claims*

NATURAL VS. SYNTHETIC

ACTIVE INGREDIENTS

SCIENTIFIC EVIDENCE

FINDING THE RIGHT PRODUCTS

FROM THE BEAUTY-OBSESSED SCIENTIST

PHYSIOLOGY FOR PRODUCTS

Let's do a quick recap of skin physiology, for products' sake.

The outermost layer of our skin is the epidermis, which endures more direct and frequent damages from the external world than any other tissue in the body. This layer is under constant assault from the sun, wind, cold, and pollution (which we all know), *and* from skincare products (the not known). Products amplify the assaults by altering the skin's acid mantel, natural moisturizing factor, microbiome, and bricks and mortar. They all get thrown out of whack by having products on them.

The skin's ability to repair and renew itself is central to its health and functioning, and certainly to its beauty. If the epidermis is destroyed (in the most severe form, a burn), we can die from dehydration. If it's just weakened, with small amounts of moisture escaping (TEWL), we will live, but our skin won't be happy or beautiful. Keeping the body's water in is vital for life. Keeping the body's water in is also vital for beauty.

Metabolically, the epidermis's most important job is to manufacture the outermost stratum corneum, both for beauty and for survival. Stratum corneum is what we see as our skin. The proper metabolism of its surface cells, corneocytes, is a prime element for aesthetically appealing skin. This layer, when healthy, protects against moisture loss and the invasion of microorganisms and pollutants.

The dermis is right below the epidermis and gives the skin hydration, suppleness, lubrication, elasticity, and a structural framework. It also houses follicles, glands, vessels, and fibers. This complex network is what supplies energy, nutrients, and water to the living epidermis. So all the good the skin needs come from *within*, not from the surface of the skin—a.k.a. products.

The epidermis renews by getting new cells from the stratum germinativum (basal) layer. A new cell takes about 30 days to go from getting *the* signal, to dividing, to arriving at the stratum corneum surface, to shedding off, and sending another signal.[113] Hence, to see any structural change on your skin, it takes at least a month. When products claim to make a difference in a week or 24 hours, you are getting a temporary masking effect on the top layer of your skin, which will go away when the product is off—it's very similar to the effects of makeup, just without the color.

While chemicals give you a temporary glow, smoothness, or evenness, they also work against your skin's structure. "What if your skin can light up the room? It can, in twenty-four hours." That's Jennifer Aniston representing Aveeno. Is she right? What is she not telling you, or does she not know herself? Skincare products will disrupt your skin's structure and functioning while Jennifer lights up the room. The best way for *your* skin to light up the room is to keep it hydrated, supple, and smooth; to ensure that its moisture barrier is working, the microbiome is balanced, and the dermis and supporting layers are regenerating in a timely manner. Products disrupt all that.

We have used skin structure (anatomy), function (physiology), product composition and effects (chemistry and biochemistry), clinical data (epidemiology), and personal testimonials (stories) to show you what healthy and beautiful skin really needs.

And we're not done yet!

COMPANIES' CLAIMS ARE TO GET YOU TO BUY

All companies making a claim about any product *should* be required to provide evidence that the product will perform as advertised. The evidence should come from scientific testing on the product itself. Unfortunately, this is not how things are done.

The first problem? Many manufacturers will use results from testing an *ingredient* in the product rather than the actual product formulation as a whole. This can be misleading because a particular ingredient can become inactive when it binds to another chemical in the formulation. Also, the ingredient may only be effective at a certain concentration or under specific conditions. Imagine if you had to decide whether a meal tasted good by sampling only one ingredient in the dish! Or, if you tried to determine whether a song sounded good by listening to just one bar of it. Sure, you could form an opinion, but it wouldn't be very well-informed.

Other manufacturers will use data that was obtained by *another* study whose results they consider favorable. However, by its very nature, that data was derived from testing done on products with completely different formulations. Cutting corners like this helps a company's bottom line more than it could possibly help protect consumers from harmful or ineffective products.

PRODUCT SAFETY

The responsibility of ensuring that a cosmetic product is safe does not fall to the FDA, as many may believe. As previously discussed, the FDA itself actually considers skincare products to be cosmetics. They are correct here! These products are temporary enhancements and cover-ups, exactly how the FDA categorized them. But skincare companies tell you they are nutrients for your skin, making you think that your skin needs them to be healthy. The opposite is true; they are in fact cosmetics. Further, this government agency only endorses that the product *probably* won't hurt you. So, FDA approval in this case actually says nothing about whether a product is efficacious, let alone effective.

Do we know many other industries where a product claims to *do something*, yet its regulatory body says *nothing* about what the product *does* and instead touts only safety? Imagine buying a car that has been approved as "safe" only to realize once you tried to drive it that the paperwork did not technically mention the vehicle could move. As a skincare product user, the first requirement on my mind is effectiveness! Being safe is just a given. If all that can be guaranteed to me is that the product is safe, and I get no assurance on its effectiveness, then why should I even bother to use it?

The burden of testing drug safety is also placed on drug manufacturers themselves, but there are some important differences. Drugs have to meet stringent requirements for safety *and* effectiveness. In the US, drugs go through both a preapproval (premarket) phase and a postapproval (postmarket) phase as long as the drug is on the market. The FDA continues to oversee the drug's safety and effectiveness as long as that drug is available to the public.[114] That's not what happens with skincare products, even though they behave very much like drugs.

These regulatory issues are not unique to the USA. In Canada, cosmetics are defined as products "used for cleaning, improving or altering the complexion, skin, hair or teeth, such as moisturizing creams, deodorants, and shampoos." Health Canada considers cosmetics self-care products alongside natural health products and nonprescription drugs.[115] However, cosmetics follow their own regulation that is different from the other two self-care categories.

First, cosmetic products can be put on the market before they receive approval. This postmarket system also means manufacturers and importers can notify Health Canada up to 10 days *after* the products have started selling. By contrast, Canada requires the other two—natural health products and nonprescription drugs—to receive premarket approval before they can be sold.

Second, during the approval process, cosmetic companies only have to provide product ingredient information, the company's contact information, and the purpose for which the cosmetic is to be used. How is product safety obtained from this? Some measure of safety is obtained from looking at the ingredient types and amounts. Given the way chemicals and ingredients interact with one another, we know a simple list is not particularly illuminating or helpful. Further, the product's actual formulation is not required to be disclosed or studied.

Third, natural health products and nonprescription drugs have to provide efficacy and quality information in addition to meeting safety standards. So, even though all three industries fall under the same Canadian Food and Drugs Act, they do not follow the same rules. Natural health products and nonprescription drugs undergo a lot more scrutiny before coming to market, while skincare products do not. And cosmetic products are not currently required to provide scientific evidence to Health Canada to support *any* claims made on the label.[116] We can only wish skincare companies would honestly say that what they are selling are cosmetics. That will be the decent heads-up for consumers.

DERMATOLOGIST TESTED

The terms "Dermatologist Tested" or "Recommended" are commonly seen on skincare products. This makes us, the consumers, feel that the product is approved and endorsed by trustworthy, knowledgeable experts. This is a very authoritative claim, and it is effective at gaining the trust of consumers. In actuality, this phrase can be used even if only one dermatologist gave the product a thumbs-up, and that "thumb" most likely was paid by the cosmetic company. It is difficult to determine how objective, unbiased, or even valid these stamps of approval could possibly be, when the conflict of interest is high.

FRAGRANCE-FREE

Before the effectiveness of a product even crosses our mind, many of us want to smell it first. If we don't like the smell, the product usually won't go into our shopping cart. That's why so many products contain fragrances.

Smells can trigger complicated memories, yet fragrance is a highly irritating substance that can also trigger severe allergic reactions. Some studies call fragrance the new secondhand smoke, citing complex compounds that are detrimental to our health.[117,118,119,120] How do skincare companies deal with this double-edged sword?

Lately, the industry has begun slapping "fragrance-free" labels on many of their products to meet this market shift. Unfortunately, the fragrance-free claim does *not* mean that fragrance was not added to the product. "Fragrance-free" simply means a complex fragrance oil—a substance usually containing a few hundred ingredients—has not been used in the product. The product can use any essential oil it wants and still be considered fragrance-free. If you are allergic to fragrances, seeking out that "fragrance-free" label will not protect you.

"Fragrance" could mean a blend of 20 or 30 different molecules. It is extremely difficult for consumers to know what product to avoid if they are allergic to fragrances. Companies understand this and are attempting to do something. If any consumer wants to know what specific fragrance ingredient is in a product, she can contact the company and they will disclose that information but with understandable delay. You won't receive an answer while you are standing in the aisle deciding whether to put the product in your cart or not. With today's instant gratification mentality, what percentage of the general public will actually bother to wait for this information to arrive and wait to buy the product?

Consumers actually want fragrance. A product that's completely without added fragrance still has a smell—an unpleasant chemical smell that's given off by the *chemicals* in the product. Even the fragrance-free shoppers don't want to smell like chemicals, so, in a way, these companies are just giving people what they want.

PRESERVATIVE-FREE

"Preservative-free" is another tricky claim. Preservatives in products are meant to kill microorganisms that spoil products and cause lotions or creams to separate or smell bad. They are essential in prolonging the shelf life of products, and are therefore highly desirable to manufacturers. While preservatives kill pathogenic organisms in products, they also kill your skin's symbiotic bacteria.

A product can be labeled "preservative-free" if it doesn't contain conventional preservatives, such as methylparaben or imidazolidinyl urea.[121] However, there are many other substances that kill microorganisms and our symbiotic bacteria. Chemicals like BHAs, AHAs, alcohols, fragrances, and essential oils all have microbe-killing power. The presence of any of these substances in a product means that product is not "preservative-free," as they can still disrupt our skin's microbiome.

If a jar of cream can last more than a week without spoiling, it's got something in it that kills something in you.

HYPOALLERGENIC

There are no FDA regulations for hypoallergenic formulas, so this term is more for marketing than for skin physiology.

COSMECEUTICAL

Cosmeceutical is a word that sounds medical, potent, and effective. The FDA offers no regulation for this term, so *anyone* can slap this claim on their product. If the product truly has medicinal benefits, then it would be a drug, not a cosmetic.

SUBJECTIVE CLAIMS

Subjective words like *look*, *feel*, and *help reduce the appearance of*, as well as self-perceptive terms like *luxurious*, *rich*, and *fresh* can make products seem enticing without actually promising anything. This kind of language, claiming something gives you "healthy-looking" skin says nothing about your skin *being* healthy. Cocaine could claim the same thing, that it makes you "happy-looking," but that says nothing about giving you a happy life. Using subjective and vague language is very effective at reducing testing requirements and curtailing regulatory or legal issues. A product that "helps reduce the appearance of fine lines" dodges a clear claim of *actually* reducing or removing unwanted lines. Skin care companies have successfully avoided being treated as drug companies and therefore avoided regulations for consumer protection.

"Olay Total Effects 7-in-1 solution. A single dose provides more Vitamin B3 than 50 cups of kale, and the formula is packed with Vitamins B3, E and C."

What an amazing claim. These nutrients sound great for our *digestive system*, but we're not supposed to eat this product. It's meant for skin. How can an organ that's designed to excrete waste absorb any of these amazing nutrients? That's if the nutrients were even there in the first place! We know the outermost layer of our skin is made up of dead cells, so how exactly are those dead cells supposed to ingest all those vitamins? This product claim contradicts skin physiology, anatomy, chemistry, biochemistry, and nature! When you put your logic hat on and block out the marketing noise, you will realize these claims are nothing but bullshit.

A 2015 study of topical skin products showed a lack of agreement between labels and the actual contents of the products.[122] Researchers examined 187 products marketed as "hypoallergenic," "for sensitive skin," "fragrance-free," "paraben-free," and "recommended by dermatologists or pediatricians" and found 167 of the 187 (89.3%) contained at least one contact allergen (a more severe form of irritants). The average number of allergens in each product was 2.4.

Product claims don't have to be proven or verified. They are nearly a free-for-all.

NATURAL VS. SYNTHETIC

The botanical trend in skin care has skyrocketed. This once niche market has grown so vast that big players are joining in. Users may feel the obligation to declare their stance as a "natural" do-gooder to show others and make themselves proud that they are health-conscious. Clearly they live a responsible life, and they know the difference between superior and inferior.

Nearly 50% of American women reportedly look for natural or organic skincare products.

Big legacy brands such as Estee Lauder and L'Oréal were slow to offer "natural" alternatives. This delay inadvertently allowed small, boutique brands to lead the way. Being ahead of the curve has kept the small players able to compete in this highly profitable industry, where big players have always dominated. In 2018, natural skincare sales totaled $1.6 billion compared to the general beauty industry, which sat at over $300 billion. The "big girls" joining the game have propelled the natural skincare market to a projected $25.11 billion by 2025.[123]

Let's again put aside the physiological fact that our skin is not designed to ingest nutrients. Would natural be better than synthetic? "Natural" conventionally means ingredients that are sourced from nature, and they are usually plant-based. For health and safety reasons, manufacturers must purify these ingredients. How much purification is enough, and how much of that process can take place before the final product is chemically altered? Suddenly, it is no longer natural.

For a long time, natural products were actually deemed problematic by cosmetic chemists. Ingredients obtained from natural sources can have inconsistent properties that depend on the amount of sun and rain they received, the places where they were harvested, and other environmental issues. Natural ingredients are very complex and can contain materials that lead to adverse reactions. M. Varinia Michalun and Joseph C. Dinardo stated:

> Using synthetic ingredients can be a way to remove unsafe impurities from natural materials, while also purifying and/or concentrating active ingredients, thereby improving quality control and yielding more effective products. There is little to nothing indicating "natural products" are more effective than those that are synthetically based. In fact, they can often be less effective. Therefore, natural versus synthetic is not really a claim relating to efficacy; it is a statement relating to lifestyle choice.

Bingo, Michalun and Dinardo!

And the botanicals (a.k.a. naturals, herbals, organics) are all complex, and many are known allergens. People who chase this "earth's natural goodness" concept tend to be those who already had a bad experience with synthetic chemicals. Either that, or they have sensitive skin. Yet some of these natural compounds are more irritating than the simpler synthetic chemicals. Here's a sample list of nature's wholesome botanicals that trigger the most irritation and allergies: *arnica, balsam, bergamot, camphor, cassia, lemon verbena, lime, marigold, menthol, sage, sandalwood, tea tree, thyme,* and *ylang-ylang.*

When it comes to products you put on your precious skin, should your pursuit be for what's natural or what's *necessary*? There are so many natural and unnatural ingredients out there, but what really matters is they are just unnecessary. You want natural? Let nature do its thing. We are not going to do better than nature. We might fool ourselves—or even nature, temporarily—but in the long run, nature is the best.

NATURAL VS. TOXIC

In pursuit of a better hair dye, I found myself thinking about using some mixture of coffee grounds, eggs, and tea. Something natural. Natural stuff would certainly be less likely to harm my body, right? With that thought, it suddenly dawned on me why people want natural products when they think of doing good things for their skin. When we think of harm, our mind goes to obviously poisonous things, like toxic chemicals. We feel that if we switch to natural materials, things that are good enough to put in our mouths—turmeric, jojoba, avocados, berries, pomegranates—then we don't have to worry about *toxicity*. If something is food-grade, it must not be bad for our skin!

Unfortunately, as we've already learned, damage does not just come from toxic or poisonous substances. Putting organic, ethically sourced, freshly squeezed lemon juice into your eyes is damaging—it's simple enough.

Placing food on our pores and assuming it won't be harmful because it's not harmful for our mouth is using the wrong logic! Your skin doesn't want food. To get nutrients into the skin from the outside, you must break down the skin's protective layers and force the substances inside through chemical actions. So, although food is much safer and better than synthetic chemicals for your digestive system, food is not good nor wanted by your skin.

When it comes to skin and skin damage, it is not just toxins, pollutants, poisons, or synthetic chemicals we need to worry about. It is disruption *to* the skin structures. Recall the extreme example of lemon juice in your eyes; most chemical substances will definitely cause irritation and disruption, but so will food! When it comes to your skin, the concern is not whether something is toxic versus edible, it is whether it will interfere with your skin's functions and if it is necessary. Raw food will irritate your skin, just like processed substances that contain surfactants, preservatives, or additives.

Our body needs good nutrients that come from *within*, through the digestive system. Whenever we interfere with this well-engineered functioning, our body will fight back with signs and symptoms. When natural substances are applied onto the skin, they cause disruptions to our skin, just like synthetic substances.

ACTIVE INGREDIENTS

It is wise to understand that if a product claims to make you look better, there had better be some active ingredients in it. However, if a product has any active ingredients, then that product is, in reality, a drug. Never use a drug long-term. Long-term drugs are for controlling symptoms and can't treat the underlying illness. A good example of this is the management of blood glucose for diabetes or taking blood pressure medication to treat hypertension. Both of these long-term drugs don't cure the underlying illnesses.

Our understanding of skincare products is decades behind that of drugs. It is time we learn that active ingredient-infused skincare products are in fact drugs. Use them like a drug to treat a specific acute problem. Correct the problem, then stop. If you use skincare products long-term, the "drug" will wreck your skin.

SCIENTIFIC EVIDENCE

Dermatologists are often asked, "Are there any moisturizers that have been proven to reduce the signs of aging?" The answer is that while moisturizer will immediately reduce the appearance of fine lines, the effect doesn't last.[124] The fine lines and wrinkles will return once the product dries out, and they will worsen. There is not a lot of scientific evidence to show that moisturizers reduce skin aging in the long term. The limited studies that have tried to prove "age-defying effects" are almost always funded by cosmetic companies, so take those "results" with a huge chunk of salt. Most of the studies with bold claims lack good clinical trials to substantiate product efficacy, and many overhyped ingredients in skincare products have *never* been shown to work from a clinical perspective.

There is also a real challenge for relying on evidence-based science, because this framework is only good for certain problems—problems that are acute; the intervention to address them is simple; and the outcome can be assessed easily and quickly.[125] In many ways, the pillar for evidenced-based medicine is infectious diseases. Infections are acute and quick to appear; the interventions are simple, like take an antibiotic; and the outcome is easy and binary to measure, such as the presence or absence of a strep throat. So, controlled trials are much simpler to conduct to gain evidence. For chronic conditions where the intervention is behavioral change, which is very complex, and the outcome is slow and progressive, it is much more complicated to control and conduct.

Beauty problems are not an acute condition (wrinkles are chronic and lasting); the intervention (the cream) is hard to isolate (what else besides the cream that has an effect on the skin); and the outcome takes a long time to confirm (immediate visual improvement that doesn't last is not an affirmative result). All these complications make it difficult to conduct valid, evidence-based skin care studies. Yet, you hear all the time that people experienced overwhelmingly positive results when using a certain cream—four out of five dermatologists approved, 80% of women had amazing results. Really?

As California plastic surgeon Dr. Zol Kryger puts it, "As honest as you want to be as a doctor, when there's money involved—when you have a vested interest in the result of a study showing something good, and you would lose money if something else comes out of it—you can't trust yourself. There's just such inherent bias in that."[126] This is another level of complication not obvious to us, but the conflict is clearly "in your face."

Several years ago at a medical conference, Dr. Elizabeth Hall Finley, a plastic surgeon from Banff, Alberta, went up to the podium and put a single slide on the projector. She didn't say a word and simply walked away. This slide was from a website called the Sunshine Act, which shows how much money every doctor in America has received from the beauty industry. This spanned income from thousands to millions of dollars.[127]

Even medical professionals are beginning to doubt the claims and results of their peers.

THE SKINCARE INDUSTRY IS NOT EVIL— NEITHER WAS SOCIAL MEDIA OR TOBACCO

I don't believe the beauty industry started their business to harm our skin. That was not their intent, just like the social media industry didn't have bad motives when it was first created. It didn't mean to control the information you could receive or your view of the world.

It did a lot of good, but it also unfortunately spun off into something that's now out of control.

When cigarettes first came out, they were not intended to give people lung cancer. The tobacco companies and farmers did not build this industry because they wanted to harm us. It took decades to collect and understand data that showed the danger of tobacco products. Whether something is helpful in the short run versus the long term takes time to discern. More importantly, it requires data to prove. Organized, unbiased, large amounts of data is necessary to show the true effects or danger of these products. In the tobacco world, that danger involves significant, long-term harm and death, so it's a lot more pressing for scientific and social forces to gather and address this life-threatening problem.

Even so, the tobacco industry fought back hard. This was because informing the public about the true nature and risks of their products would certainly result in a substantial monetary loss. Remember, *doctors* used to publicly endorse their favorite brands of tobacco products. The tobacco industry may not have wanted to give people cancer, but they did want to sell cigarettes.

Money makes things complicated. Companies have stockholders to answer to and quarterly profits to meet. Eventually, the original vision—creating products that are good for people—gets blurred.

In the case of the cosmetic and skincare industry, itchy skin, dry patches, fine lines, a little sensitivity, and acne are such minor problems when compared to something like lung cancer. Also, the profits are humongous and people like the look, smell, and feel of the products. So where's the incentive for anyone, including many of the handsomely paid scientist consultants, to reveal the product's *long-term* health and beauty risks?

The beauty industry is not an evil entity. It just stands to make a lot of money from us and will make a whole lot more if we don't know their products are harming us.

FINDING THE RIGHT PRODUCTS

For each of you who have chased the best *product* for your skin, have you ever thought that the pursuit should be for the best "care," rather than "product"? Our default position has always involved products—a race among products to see which one most fits your unique skin. Water was never in the running. Put simply, water is the best "product" for your skin. Drinking water and gently cleaning with water is really all we need. Not many people believe that water alone is enough, let alone the best choice. Water is truly clean, sustainable, inclusive, and kind. Products have been in our lives for too long, and each product creates the need for another. This vicious cycle has made water appear outclassed and insufficient.

If the product you use works, then why do you eventually need to add a night cream, a day serum, an exfoliant, a mask, an overnight elixir, spa treatments, and more? Aging alone does not create so many issues that we need a counter full of products to keep things under control.

There is no magical way for your skin to always look great, not even with *Skin Sobering*. Your skin is alive, and it is affected by how you live. As your lifestyle changes, so will your skin. Give your body some time to adjust, and allow it to return to its natural equilibrium without chemical help.

10

LIFESTYLE

HOW YOU LIVE AFFECTS HOW YOU LOOK

SMOKING

SUN

DIET

EAST VS. WEST, WET VS. DRY

GENETICS

EXERCISE

POLLUTION

FROM THE BEAUTY-OBSESSED SCIENTIST

Skin Sobering is a lifestyle. It is a way of living that encourages you to fuss less on things nature is already taking care of and do more to build your immune system and well-being. If you didn't want to or couldn't bother to change anything else in your life, the discontinuation of fussy skincare products is the simplest and most effective way to improve your skin's health and beauty. Anything else is much harder to change than the simple act of dropping the hassle of putting on and taking off skincare products.

SMOKING

Smoking is all harm and no benefits. It is the worst enemy to beauty and health. Teenagers may be trading a couple of pounds (if any) for bad breath, stained teeth, and dry, sallow, wrinkled skin. How good-looking is a smoker's face? A yellowing of the skin as a result of sped-up glycation can rear its ugly head as early as a person's 30s. The money and time spent on cigarettes to lose the 2 pounds could be much better spent dragging yourself outside or to the gym.

Smoking increases oxidation (free-radical formation) in the skin and body. Smokers have fewer antioxidants (free-radical fighters) in their skin than nonsmokers. Since smokers lack the antioxidants to fight back against the oxidation smoking brings them, they can experience some severe signs of glycation, like discolored skin, wrinkles, sagginess, and loss of radiance.

Further, nicotine causes the blood vessels in your heart, lungs, and skin to constrict, decreasing capillary blood flow to your skin. This robs it of nourishment and releases more free radicals. In time, the reduced blood supply thins all three skin layers and causes your skin to be permanently leathery and wrinkled. It's an ugly look, as simple as that.

AUDREY'S CIGARETTE HOLDER

What's the most vivid image in your mind when you think of the elegant Ms. Audrey Hepburn? Mine is her bateau neckline little black dress, long satin gloves, baby bangs with a high bun, and the skinny cigarette holder. That look is so iconic that, lacking any one of those elements just isn't the *Hepburn look*. Hepburn smoked at Tiffany's and in real life. It was said that she sometimes smoked up to three packs a day,[128] yet to so many, Hepburn was and is a paragon of poise, elegance, and grace that few American actresses can measure up to. Um...that's not good for the public health image, and perhaps it is one of the reasons responsible for the difference in skin conditions between Asian and Western women?[129]

The American Lung Association reported that 13.5% of African American women smoke. That number rises to 16% of Non-Hispanic Whites and 24% of Native American women. Only 2.6% of Asian American women smoke. Other reports show a similar pattern, where the percentage of White women who smoke is about 20%, whereas Chinese and Korean women's smoking rate is in the low single digits.[130] These are huge differences, and we know what smoking does to collagen and elastin! If you smoke, your skin is going to turn ugly much sooner, even for a beauty like Audrey Hepburn.

SUN

The major difference between skin that looks old and skin that looks young is the extent of sun exposure it has endured. We hope you are more than familiar with the sun's effects on your skin. If not, ultraviolet light (UVA and UVB) in the sun's rays can give you a scorching sunburn and prematurely aging skin. We feel sunburns right away, but photoaging and skin cancer are more subtle and destructive. These only show up after long-term exposure.

Photoaging refers to sun damage that happens when UV light from the sun or tanning beds hits your unprotected skin and causes damage to its structure. Photodamage happens in the deep layers of the skin, so it can take years before the signs become visible to the naked eye. These signs are wrinkling, hyperpigmentation, loss of skin elasticity, roughness, unevenness, broken capillaries, redness, and blotchiness.

For simplicity and so you can remember this easily, UVA is responsible for *Aging*. UVB causes *Burns* and precancerous cells. Both are bad for your skin's beauty and health. It is now recognized that although UVA and UVB are responsible for 90% of photoaging, high-energy visible light (HEV) and infrared light accounts for the remaining 10%.[131] HEV, also known as blue light, comes from the sun and from screens, like smartphones and tablets. Infrared light is invisible to the eye, but it can be felt as heat.

We need the sun for Vitamin D and for day-to-day life. Sun is energy, and sun is happiness, but we don't need to use our face to receive these rays. Let the much larger areas of your arms and legs get the required amount of sunshine, and protect your face from solar damage.

SPF

SPF stands for "Sun Protection Factor." For a product that has an SPF of 15, it means the time it takes for UVB exposure to burn your skin is extended by 15 times. So, if it normally takes your skin 10 minutes to burn, applying an SPF 15 sunscreen will enable you to stay in the sun for 150 minutes without burning if the sunscreen was properly applied and didn't come off. Skin burning is instantly visible and felt, so it brings immediate attention. We are more careful about preventing burns than photoaging.

UVA, on the other hand, is a quiet but powerful thief. There are roughly 500 times more UVA rays in sunlight than UVB. UVA steals your skin's beauty slowly and surely. It doesn't burn the skin like UVB, so people can forget that damage is still taking place while you are preventing burns. UVA is the biggest contributor to aging skin, yet the term *SPF* gives no protection indication for UVA at all. So, you may be able to extend your no-burn exposure with UVB protection, but UVA is still penetrating deep inside your skin. That cumulative, irreversible damage will appear sooner or later! Sneaky!

It was not until 2012 that government labeling regulations began to use the term "broad-spectrum" or put a UVA symbol on sunscreen bottles to indicate UVA protection.[132] That's a start, but there's still no degree of protection specified for UVA. In Japan, there's a UVA protection rating system called PA, which is converted from a PPD (persistent pigment darkening) rating system. PA+ indicates low UVA protection, PA++ indicates moderate UVA protection, and PA+++ indicates high UVA protection.[133]

To balance the damaging effects of skincare products—including sunscreen, photoaging, and the life-giving goodness of the sun, follow these sun protection tips:

- **Best**—Avoid the sun on your face and use physical protection like shade, an umbrella, a wide-brim hat, a face mask, and sunglasses. You are not avoiding living, just avoiding UV on your face.

- **Good**—If you are exposed to the sun for more than 15 minutes straight, use physical sunscreen that contains zinc oxide and titanium dioxide only, with a mineral powder or petroleum base. Don't stare at your screen endlessly. Cut down. I use blue light shields on screens to lower HEV exposure to my eyes and skin.

- **Okay**—Use chemical sunscreen containing mainly UVB-absorbing chemical ingredients. It is better than exposing your bare face to the sun for more than 15 minutes. Chemical sunscreen, however, contains all the skin-harming ingredients. Wash it off as soon as you are not outdoors.

- **Worst**—No protection at all, bearing your face to the sun for hours, and using tanning beds!

DIET

For great skin and health, work from within! Eat real food, not too frequently, enjoy it—especially plants (inspired by Michael Pollan's simpler, seven-word phrase: *Eat food, not too much, mostly plants*)!

Eating well affects your health, and that shows up on your skin. There were long-held beliefs in dermatology that diet didn't have much to do with the skin, but many recent studies show that what you eat is the most important factor in your health, including how your skin looks.[134] Acne is exacerbated by sugar, refined carbohydrates, and dairy. This is because of increasing insulin levels and inflammation. A great complexion is aided by omega-3 fatty acids and dietary fiber.[135] This is not news, and it is gaining new strength in the modern Western medical world. In fact, our digestive system, the condition of our gut, and our gut's microbiome have everything to do with our health and skin. Many forms of skin disorders—acne, rosacea, psoriasis, eczema, and premature wrinkling, are now believed to be expressions of inflammation and irregularities in the gut.[136]

GLYCATION

There are many more connections between food and your skin. Sugar itself is bad for the skin. Sugar, in combination with heat and animal protein, is a different level of bad—in the form of glycation. Glycation (which is similar to the Maillard reaction in the browning of foods) is a process where sugar molecules attach themselves to the amino acids in collagen and elastin proteins.[137] These proteins are the structural makeup of the dermis and are what make your skin youthful, plump, and springy. The more sugars in your diet, the more glycation occurs. Sugars tangle with protein fibers, causing the skin to look stiff, saggy, discolored, and wrinkly.

The process of glycation, like free-radical formation and inflammation, occurs naturally in the human body as a product of a normal metabolism. Still, what we eat can slow down or accelerate these skin-aging processes. High heat, dry cooking methods with the presence of sugar, refined carbohydrates, or dairy increase the rate of glycation both in the food and in our body. Foods that have been grilled, fried, roasted, baked, broiled, or barbecued promote glycation. Glycation also triggers more free radical formation, oxidative stress, and inflammation, all of which make the skin look bad.

In the late stages of the glycation process of high-heat cooking, advanced glycation end products (AGEs—apropos) are formed in the food.[138] When ingested, these cause further inflammation. Consuming foods cooked with the aforementioned high-heat methods can increase your total daily AGEs intake by 25%. AGEs intake subsequently accelerates your body's own production of AGEs.[139] The presence of AGEs also makes your skin more vulnerable to other negative factors, such as UV rays and cigarette smoke. Besides making the skin look old, AGEs also play a detrimental role in hardening blood vessels and twisting nerves, causing further damage, such as kidney disease, diabetes, vascular diseases, and cognitive decline.

Interestingly, herbs and spices like ginger, garlic, and cinnamon can inhibit glycation, as can consuming raw foods.

ORGANIC FOODS AND PRODUCTS

When it comes to eating well, there's still a debate surrounding organic food. Organic food likely adds value to those who are doing most things well already, like eating a plant-abundant diet, exercising regularly, sleeping well, managing stress effectively, not smoking or doing drugs, and not drinking excessively. If they are doing all of that, then eating organic foods may add that extra 5% boost to their overall health.

On the other hand, people who regularly consume fast food, soda, and refined carbs might have a different experience. Add to that, if they prefer vegging on their couch to putting veggies in their mouth, their body is probably only functioning at about 30%. Adding a 5% improvement with organic, non-GMO, locally sourced, or grain-fed expensive foods is not going to do much for you. Thirty-five percent is still failing. Change your big habits first instead of fussing over the minor details.

There is no debate that fruits and vegetables are good for our digestive system, but these same, beneficial foods are not good to put on our skin. A lot of marketing muscles falsely attach food values to skin care principles in an effort to try to convince us we should spend more money to get the "better" products. Remember that organic or not, products are not what our skin wants on its surface. Essential oils and their fragrances are as natural as they claim to be, but they are also among some of the most allergenic and irritating substances out there when it comes to skin. "Natural" does not automatically mean "healthy" or "beneficial." So those "organic friends of the earth" who opt for natural skincare products to do good for the world might as well go truly natural and organic—just use water. The world will be much better off without all the bottles and the processing that goes into making them.

FOOD AND ITS BROKEN NUTRIENTS

There's a joke about food and culture I heard somewhere and have told many times, and it goes like this: Japanese people eat with their eyes—the black plate, pink salmon, yellow tuna, green seaweed, and white daikon; colors, shapes, sizes that are harmonized beautifully and presented in perfection. The French eat with their hearts—the violin, candlelight, ambiance, a room with a view, and food prepared with love. British people eat with their noses (as in snobbishness, sorry)—etiquette, table manners, dress codes, cutlery rules, dishes rules, serviette rules, and body posture rules. North Americans eat with their brains—counting calories, weighing carbs, analyzing proteins and fats, and dissecting macronutrients and micronutrients. Here comes the last one, if the above haven't been stereotyping enough. Chinese eat with their taste buds—it doesn't matter if there are cockroaches on the floor, flies in the air, the waitstaff is rude and spitting away, you having to share a table with strangers, or whether there are eyes, heart, brain, tongue, ears, intestines, fallopian tubes, knuckles, feet, and plant scraps served on your plate, as long as the food tastes good, the Chinese will line up to chow down. But we don't eat the nose. That's barbaric, gross!

Jokes aside, there are things we can learn from each other's cultures. In some cultures, food is a relationship rather than energy and nutrients. Too many people, especially North Americans, think of food primarily as a vehicle to deliver nutrition. According to Dr. Marion Nestle, professor of nutrition, that "takes the nutrient out of the context of food, the food out of the context of diet, and the diet out of the context of lifestyle." To eat well is to enjoy the food itself, and not to worry about the individual nutrients in it. Eating well is also not an indulgence, not an escape, and definitely not a convenient fix for boredom. Eating well is eating real and whole foods as part of socializing. It should be a medium to human interaction and personal pleasure. Cook your own meals as much as possible, and grow or raise your own food if at all possible. When we have a good relationship with food, it is joy, not broken-down nutrients or guilt.

Conversely, when we look at food as individual nutrients, we render ourselves unable to see the forest for the trees. Journalist and activist Michael Pollan expressed this better than I can:

> Researchers have found, based on epidemiological comparisons of different populations, that a diet high in fruits and vegetables confers some protection against cancer. So naturally they ask, "What nutrients in those plant foods are responsible for that effect?" One hypothesis is that the antioxidants in fresh produce—compounds like beta carotene, lycopene, vitamin E, etc.—are the X factor. It makes good

sense: these molecules (which plants produce to protect themselves from the highly reactive oxygen atoms produced in photosynthesis) vanquish the free radicals in our bodies, which can damage DNA and initiate cancers. At least that's how it seems to work in the test tube. Yet as soon as you remove these useful molecules from the context of the whole foods they're found in, as we've done in creating antioxidant supplements, they don't work at all. Indeed, in the case of beta carotene ingested as a supplement, scientists have discovered that it actually increases the risk of certain cancers. Big oops. [140]

Nature is full of amazing things, but we need to use and consume them in their natural and whole form, otherwise the benefits are questionable. Whole wheat without bran and germ is just refined white flour, with many of its proteins lost. Brown rice with its hull milled away becomes refined white rice that lacks bran and thiamine. Fiber in food versus fiber extracted and added back to something else functions totally differently, making its benefits debatable. Coupled with heavy processing, these extracted compounds have gone through a complete reformation and consequently their nutrients are lost.

How then and why do consumers trust processed foods? Manufacturers add ingredients and make *claims* to justify the existence of these refined products. Sugary cereals scream about their whole grain goodness, along with enhanced vitamins and fortified nutrients. Some packaging even suggests these products could save us from heart attacks. Creams and lotions declare their miracles as well, with added Vitamin C, E, B, A, retinols, ceramides, hyaluronic acid, AHAs, peptides, and more. Of course, they claim this fancy enrichment will take years off of your face. Real foods over in the apple and the broccoli aisle don't talk like processed cereals do, and no claims are made about your tap water. Why is that? Real, natural things that are truly good for you don't need packages, and they don't have big budgets.

In his book *In Defense of Food*, Michael Pollan wrote, "The quieter the food, likely the healthier the food." This applies to skin care as well. The more claims these companies shout out, the more desperate they are to get us to buy their products. Also remember, when nutrients are broken off of their naturally existing form, they don't behave the same. Even if our skin could eat or absorb Vitamins ABCDEFG for long-term benefits, what's in the bottle is not the right version. Skincare products are like packaged foods in that both are fun to use or consume on occasion but are harmful if they become daily fare.

EAST VS. WEST, WET VS. DRY

When it comes to body constitution, is there an "ours is better than yours" situation between Eastern and Western skin? There is an obvious difference in color among races, but is one group more genetically blessed than the other, with porcelain texture, plumpness, and fewer wrinkles? Or are there some other factors? Though I will be making generalizations just to emphasize some points, I am also very aware that there are as many differences within a group (meaning among Chinese people themselves) as there are between groups (between Chinese and Caucasian, Black, and Hispanic, etc.). The differences among people are more due to how they live and behave than their race.

Some articles attribute the East and West skin differences to Asians having a thicker dermis. The idea here is Asians must have more collagen and elastin, so they have fewer wrinkles. Is Asian skin genetically blessed? I would think if it is, we would notice that Western babies and children have less supple, less plump, and less pinchable cheeks. Well, that's just not the case. Both Eastern and Western babies (and Southern and Northern and Central—all babies) are born with beautiful and lovable skin. So, when "studies" say that the Asian dermis is thicker, is that a reflection of Asian genetics or of

Asian lifestyle? This is yet another incarnation of the age-old "nature versus nurture" argument.

WET VS. DRY

While we are still discussing the effects of food, let's examine the way how and what we eat makes a difference to our skin. When Westerners see that Asians have a smooth and firm complexion, or when Easterners see that Caucasians have a fair and rosy color, we immediately attribute these characteristics to the most convenient explanation: genetics. Then we seek what they use, because we have been conditioned to hope there is magic in a bottle to change how we look.

You are what you eat. This is an overused but true cliché. The world's cuisines differ from one another in so many ways, and there are countless write-ups and cookbooks that tell these tales. That said, I haven't come across many that dissect the world's cuisines the way I'm thinking of them: dry versus wet. I believe this difference is a significant contributor to and differentiator of skin beauty between the East and the West.

Let's look at the ways we cook. Of course, nowadays our cooking methods and preferences intersect and overlap. After all, we are a global culture, and we have easy access to each other's culinary arts. Still, there is a noteworthy fondness that's predominant in these two cultures respectively (please pardon me for oversimplifying the East and the West). When it comes to North American cooking, I've observed there's a much higher frequency of baking, frying, deep-frying, grilling, roasting, broiling, searing, braising, and barbecuing. These well-loved Western cooking methods produce crispy, crunchy, smoky, golden, caramelized, and crusty foods. These textures may be much preferred in the West, but just spell D-R-Y to me and my peeps. These are not the go-to cooking options for most Asians.

The more frequently employed cooking methods in Chinese cuisines are steaming, stewing, sautéing, simmering, boiling, blanching, and even finer distinctions in some of them that don't translate well into English, like 煲, 燉, 煮, 蒸, 燙, 滾, 燜, 煨, 涮, 氽, 焯, 灼, 泡, 焓, 滷, 淥, 溜. We have three times the number of slow-low cooking methods than the English vocabulary can describe. These are all "wet" cooking methods that give food a texture of sticky, slimy, chewy, mushy, gelatinous, glutinous, slurpy, gooey, squishy, slippery, wet, moist, rubbery, tendony—Mmmm! These heavenly, lip-smacking textures sound revolting to my husband and kids but are loved by all my people. *Bland-steamed chicken* 白切雞 (bai zhan ji; free-range, yellow-skin, firm-muscle chicken, steamed or dipped in boiling water) is one of the old-time favorites in Chinese cuisine. How night and day different is that compared to the all-famous Western fried chicken? We even prefer peanuts—a common crunchy, roasted food in the West—boiled and wet! Yum, yum!

At my Sunday family brunches, the kids and I constantly fight over who gets to cook the bacon. They find my meaty, chewy, and moist pieces uncooked and lame, whereas I think their crunchy, snappable strips are no different than salted tree bark that will just give me a sore throat (this is a Traditional Chinese Medicine [TCM] thing, 熱氣 (re qi), or "inner heat" caused by high-heat, dry cooking). The difference is even applied to desserts. Consider baked goods versus fruits; cookies and pies versus mochis and sweet soups. This is dry versus wet yet again.

While North Americans love a good cut of muscle meat and the costly white breast, we Asians fight for the marrow, brain, maw, belly, knuckle, feet, tongue, and brown meat. These are all pricey delicacies in our markets. In this, Asians are not unique. Europeans love their traditional survival foods as well. Take garum, a strong relish made of rotten fish guts loved by rich Romans in ancient times, or the French bouillabaisse, a stew made by Marseille fishermen using fish bones, heads, skin, and shellfish scraps. These are as wet and whole as you can get. Waste-averse cultures consume the way they do because people eat what is available, and they learn to put together a sumptuous diet that supports life and conservation. These cultures survived and these diets thrived for longevity and skin beauty.

What do all these wet-cooking methods boil down to? Less glycation! If Chinese people do have firmer, plumper, and more supple skin, it may have more to do with what we eat and how we cook. For beauty's sake, pay attention to how often you are using high-heat, dry cooking methods.

EAT THE PART TO NOURISH THE PART

We Chinese don't stop there. We have another thing: *eat the part to nourish the part* 以型補型 (yi xing bu xing). Chinese people from my region eat cooked animal brains because they believe it will make them smarter. They also eat feet thinking it will improve mobility. These parts are quite tasty, if you found a good way to cook them when you were forced to eat all parts of an animal to avoid starvation—including testicles, penis, and labia. Now, I bet a lot of animal genitals are consumed by the Chinese not because of starvation, but because some men think consuming these parts will make their own genitals more potent.

A load of crap, isn't it? Well, the idea that putting hyaluronic acid *on* your skin because your skin has hyaluronic acid *inside* it is just as ridiculous.

Eating body parts and believing that part will enhance your part, and putting acid on your face and thinking it will transform to what your skin needs are not exactly the same belief, but they are equally moronic. At least animal testicles and penises are a great source of protein and fat, perfectly fine pieces of meat from nature. But trying to get hyaluronic acid, ceramide, niacinamide, retinol, Vitamin C or E through the surface of our impermeable skin? It is antinature! Our skin has all these compounds in it, all of which are required for the skin to stay youthful. However, you can only get these nutrients to your skin by eating real foods that contain these substances. Even so, nobody can guarantee that these nutrients are going to go to your skin. They will go where your body chooses to send them.

When you ingest fat, it doesn't go straight to your boobs or booty to plump them up, nor does it skip your midriff to keep your waistline small. Most of us know by now that when we try to lose fat, we can't target a specific area at the exclusion of others. It is naïve to think that we can control where the fat goes, and it is equally gullible to believe the impermeable barrier of our skin will allow substances like hyaluronic acid to do the job nature designed our skin to do on its own. The notion this could happen without resulting in any bad effects is ignorance.

A HEALTHY DIET

A lot of foodies who claim they will eat anything declare that texture is their final frontier. A squishy, slippery, rubbery, and chewy texture will be what stops them from enjoying many wet-cooked foods. Disliking these wet textures is not really the diet roadblock to health it may appear to be. What is more problematic with North American eating is the lack of a healthy diet in general.

According to Michael Pollan, a healthy diet consists of eating almost anything as long as the food is varied and you don't eat too much of it too frequently. Unfortunately, the North American diet is not varied.[141] Canadian-American longevity physician Peter Attia calls it the "Standard American Diet" or SAD. Most of the plants North Americans rely on are grains, not leaves. Corn, soybeans, wheat, and rice account for two-thirds of the calories North Americans consume. Considering there are 3,000 nutritious plants to choose from, overconsumption of these four crops represents a worrisome, unhealthy simplification of the food web.[142]

Further, in much of the world, the ratio of meat and fresh vegetables is also completely different than the distorted proportions of SAD. Most cultures use meat or protein sparingly, almost as a flavoring or garnish. Vegetables are the main food group offered, not a "side dish" garnishing a 16-ounce hunk of meat as we see in North America. People from cultures where they consume less meat live much longer and are healthier. What you eat clearly has an impact on how well you are going to live and what your body looks like.

A final note on food in loving memory of my favorite food storyteller, Anthony Bourdain. When he interviewed French-American chef and culinary educator Jacques Pépin, Bourdain asked, "So, what do you think of this whole gluten problem?" Pépin's cavalier answer was that he'd never heard of it. The chef went on to explain that when he was young, a food problem meant not having enough or that it didn't taste good. When he was growing up, there were almost no food allergies. Pépin then said the problem with food allergies are processed foods and chemicals. People are just eating too many nonfoods, and their bodies do not know what to do other than to start rejecting things. The goal may be to reject things it specifically doesn't like, but because these chemicals are tied up in food itself, the body eventually rejects bad food, real food, and beyond food.

The same is happening with skin allergies—chemicals. That includes the so-called "natural" skincare products that are, in reality, highly processed.

BEACH AND BLEACH

Now another beauty crime and another big difference between the East and the West: our love and hate of the sun. Asian women don't want to have freckles, and they definitely don't want to look dark. They avoid the sun like the plague. They slather sunscreen on their faces day and sometimes even night (night sunscreen is for protection from fluorescent light, my goodness!). They wrap their faces in balaclavas during summer and winter outdoor activities, wear masks and tinted "welder mask" sun visors (long before COVID-19) to block UV rays, not germs. Umbrella use is prevalent. Golfers swing more than their clubs, soccer moms obstruct other spectators, and shoppers poke out the eyes of other pedestrians, all of them with their umbrellas fully open under a clear blue sky. I own many umbrellas and save them for sunny days.

Then there are these viral images of Chinese and Korean women wearing condom-like, head-face-neck swim gear on the beach (Ellen DeGeneres calls it a "face-kini"). It slips on one's head and neck just like a condom on the penis, with the difference of the four built-in holes for seeing and breathing. This is not an urban legend, and those images were not staged to gain likes on social media. They are candid shots of real-life beachwear. I am not obsessed enough to own one.

So, for the less obsessed like me, we will walk under shaded areas, use an umbrella, wear a hat, put on a mask, and are never caught outside without high SPF sunscreen if we really can't shield our face in any other way. Here are some pictures of me cycling, skiing, reading, and driving. When I first started cycling with a mask nine years ago, people thought I was a deviant. As they got to know me, I was upgraded to "strange." My bubbly personality grew on them, and I became "quirky." Last year, they thought I was "cute," and now that we are friends, I am this adorable "cover" girl who hides her face from the sun.

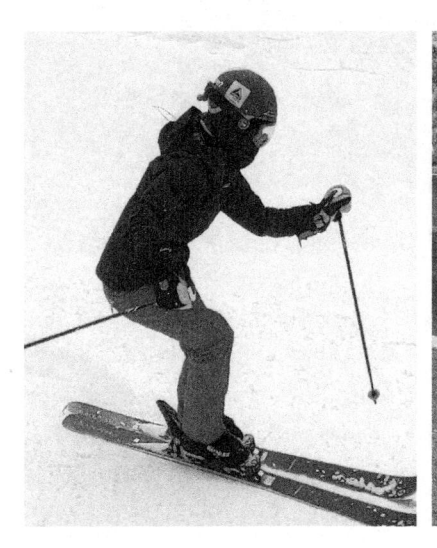

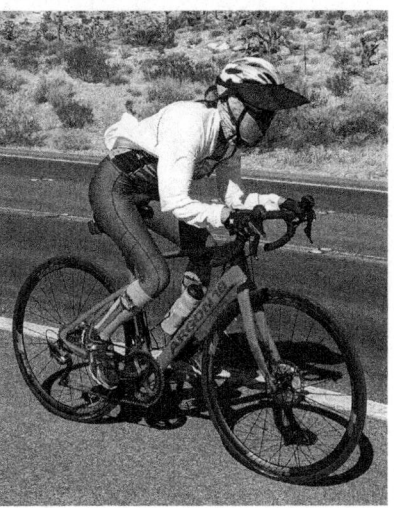

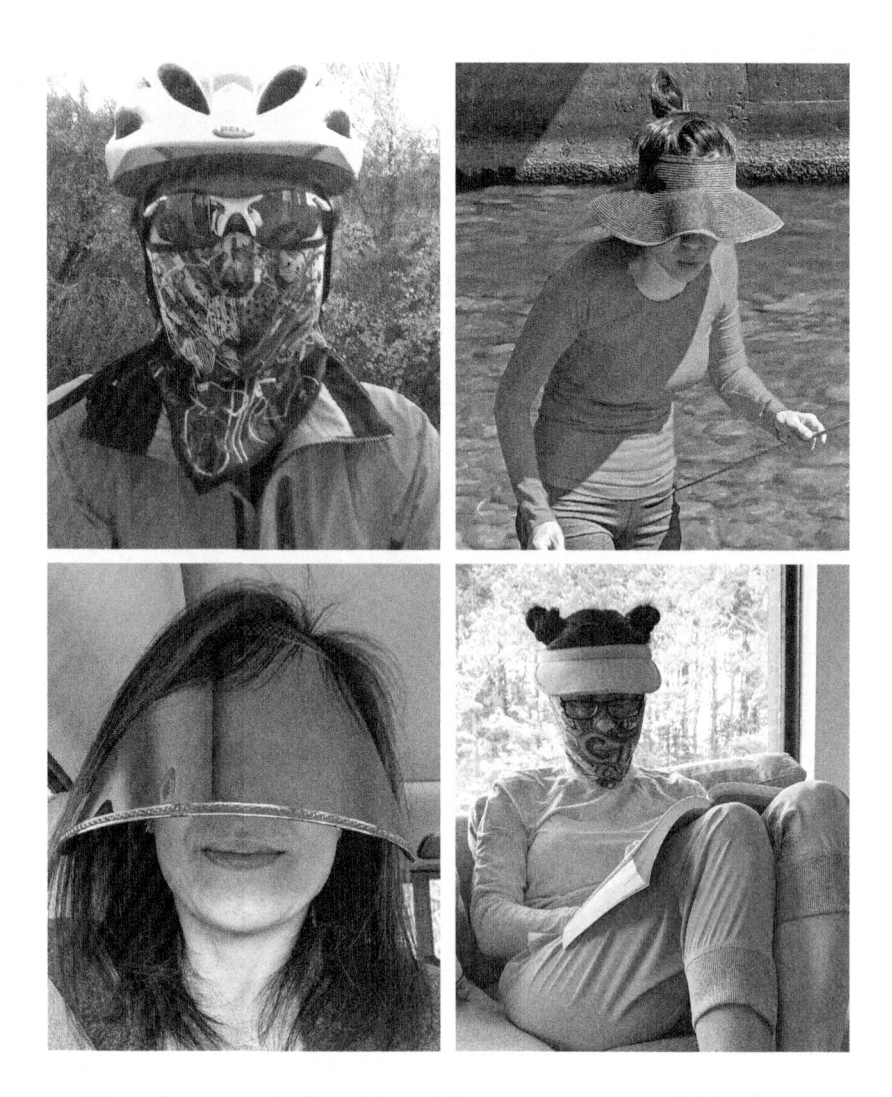

What do naturally fair-skinned Western women do? Their culture is different, and they want to get some color. In the West, looking pale is synonymous with working a cubical, no-window, sedentary job. Conversely, a tan signifies health, free time, and adventurousness. The fact that the sun causes aging is less of a concern to them, as its consequential harm is not immediate. Achieving a tan is appealing and an instant gratification. If their skin doesn't burn easily, many Westerners will skip the sunscreen. Photoaging likely skipped their mind too.

It takes decades for accelerated aging caused by exposure to the sun to show up. You won't see much of that in your 20s and 30s, but once you do start to see it, the damage has already been done. You can almost word-for-word apply the same benefits and harms to skincare products. So, Western women's skin problems like wrinkles and sagginess are not because they are "children of a lesser god." Rather, this is due to protein loss from sun exposure and likely high-heat cooking as well.

Asian women have a much lower prevalence of photoaging, but we (and other East and South Asians) have another problem. We dislike being dark so much that we bleach our skin. Beauty-obsessed and even regular Asians have almost all used some form of bleaching cream on their face to help whiten that yellow tone. It's called 美白 (mei bai)—*white-beautifying*. As a result, skin loses its luster and the tone is replaced by more shades of gray. That was me once, and the only way to save my looks (not skin) was layers of dewy-colored paints called foundation. Asian women's skin may be supple and plump from sun avoidance, but it is also thin and sensitive from product use.

In pursuit of these colors that we were not born with, Eastern and Western people voluntarily seek the greatest damaging methods: sun and hydroquinone; beach and bleach.

It seems both Westerners and Easterners have a relationship with the sun that doesn't seem to be health-oriented. Instead, it is more a matter of color preference. It may be hard to recondition people to appreciate every color of skin or even their own skin, sadly. However, the agreed-upon subjective measures of *beautiful* skin—clear, smooth, radiant, glowing, plump, taut, supple, firm—are actually the universal standard of *healthy* skin as well. This is achievable by universally changing our skin health understanding and behavior.

You've already been introduced to this. It is called *Skin Sobering*.

The Influence of the East

The Korean double-cleanse method is endorsed by so many people in the West. Alexandria Ocasio-Cortez, an outspoken American politician, swears by it. The method involves a first-round clean with an oil-based cleanser, which is intended to break down and remove stubborn impurities like skin cream, makeup, silicones, and sunscreen, followed by a water-based cleanser to wash off the first cleanser.

Ocasio-Cortez was in her 20s when she made that double-cleanse statement. That is very young skin, supposedly vibrant skin. Did she need that kind of cleansing, or is she the prodigal product of a product-obsessed culture who inadvertently made her skin bad through diligent product use? If she has replaced her own oil, a natural moisturizer, with the synthetic oil of processed lotions, she has taken away her precious natural luminosity. Which is worse, her own oil or chemical oil? And the worst, she can't wash away synthetic oil with warm water. She has to use chemical cleansers. And why use oil-based makeup? Because it has great coverage to hide damage and flaws. Again, Alexandria was in her 20s! How much damage had she incurred from intrinsic skin aging (chronological) versus extrinsic assaults from products, environment, and lifestyle?

When extrinsic damage is reduced through *Skin Sobering*, the skin will regain its dewiness and smoothness. This makes mineral powder makeup enough to brighten your face and even out your tone if needed.

Despite all the wrong messages spread by the East, they are serious about sun protection and not smoking, and those are the right messages to spread. I believe that's the main reason you see so much good in Korean women's skin, despite all the product harm they've put it through. They have zero sun damage.

According to the American Cancer Society, skin cancer is the most common cancer, accounting for almost 50% of all cancers in the United States. However, in sun-fearing South Korea, skin cancer doesn't even make their top 10 list of common cancers. Sun avoidance is practiced among people young and old, women and men. Korean people also believe in the health benefits of fermented foods. Kimchi is a must for each meal, which is great for the skin.

South Korea also has the highest per capita rate of plastic surgeries in the world, meaning that many Koreans have augmented faces. People who have had botched surgeries tend not to show themselves off, so we mainly see only the successful ones. The fancy statistical term for this is "selection bias," and it is pretty clear that this is partly why we see so many images of beautiful Koreans. It is also common knowledge that Korean people invest a lot in other clinical procedures like lasers, peels, and injections to remove long-term skin damage. Culturally, Korean women also feel a duty to put their best made-up face forward, so they learn how to use makeup skillfully and diligently.

When your skin is not exposed to UV rays, you don't smoke, and you eat well, you have done your skin a huge favor, and you can afford to commit a few skin *product* crimes without paying too high of a price—yet. When you invest a ton of time, money, and learning into looking beautiful, you will look mighty fine as long as you are all dressed up and made up, especially in electronic images. Once the products are off, is your skin really better?

GENETICS

Genetics is king, but when we take personal responsibility and examine our lifestyle, we see plenty of evidence that what we do determines much more of our health and beauty than what we can blame on our ancestors. Inversely, if we abuse our genetic gifts, the early winners can end up as losers.

We compare ourselves to others, even if we don't discuss it aloud. Perhaps you remember the girl in your grade school who had beautiful skin, or your friend in junior high with a smooth, poreless complexion.

That's their genetics. Some people's skin is just better looking than others (based on the culturally defined social metrics). We cannot change our genetics. But while I am jealous of Lan's skin, I know I have strengths in other traits. Accept the (skin) card that you were dealt and make the best of it. The main difference going forward is how you play those cards. Lan rarely uses skincare products, and she admittedly is too lazy to do more than just wash with water. I should've copied her, and I wish I had known better.

We can't coast on good genes for too long, especially if we don't have the right knowledge to make them benefit us. I was a skinny girl with the preferred body type for Asians. I didn't have to do much to stay thin, and I ate like a horse. I was just genetically lucky. When I was 9, my cousin said, "Kid, watch out. If you eat like this, you'll get fat when you reach adulthood. All the Tjams get fat." At 17, I was still a skinny girl. My cousin announced again, "Girl, don't be cocky. You'll get fat when you get married. All Tjam women do." At 26, I got married and fit into a size small dress. At my wedding, that same cousin said, "Well, wait till you have kids. Most people get fat after kids." Three boys later, I went from a size six to a two (that's a fashion industry sizing trick. I didn't actually shrink, but the point remains). I continued to eat more than some men I knew.

Then, my cousin cast this final curse, "Wait till menopause. No one can escape that." And bingo! Almost. In my early 40s, my weight started to climb, and it reached a level I couldn't stand. My genetic advantage was beaten by the cruel reality of aging and hormones, and most crucially, my horse-like appetite.

Fast forward seven years. Bruce and I learned all we could about food, fasting, fitness, and longevity. We read books and learned from reputable scientific sources, and I am finally back to my 17-year-old waistline. I no longer have the genetic advantage, but persistently doing healthy things allowed me to overcome my cousin's prophecy. Bruce and I still have massive amounts of enjoyment with sumptuous, real foods. And at every available opportunity, I make my dearest cousin Hardy—the food lover and big spender—treat me big time. And he is, as always, loving and teasing.

Even the genetically underprivileged can win the long march by doing what's right for their bodies. If you don't learn how to play the cards you're dealt, genetics will eventually fail you too. With the right information and good health behaviors, time will tell who's the tortoise and who's the hare.

EXERCISE

Exercise is great for your health but not so efficient for weight loss. If you were ever discouraged by exercise not slimming your figure quickly enough, I hope this will reenergize you.

In 2014, Dr. Mark Tarnopolski of McMaster University published a study that examined the relationship between skin, aging, and exercise.[143] He found that active, exercising mice aged slower, had less wrinkled skin, and less gray fur. The experiment was repeated with humans between 20 and 84 years old. Results showed that as participants got older, their skin thickness and elasticity was reduced *except* for those who exercised. Exercising is not just a good lifelong goal; it also has a protective effect against aging!

In order to rule out other confounding factors (diet, smoking, sleep, and genetics), the study was repeated with a group of people ages 65 and older who didn't exercise. These subjects were assigned a moderate program of aerobic exercise for 30 minutes, twice weekly. After three months, their skin had changed dramatically. Their stratum corneum, epidermis, and dermis resembled those of people between 20 and 40 years old. This remarkable change was measured in the participants' buttocks to rule out sun and natural elements effects—a cheeky research design.

Those of you inspired by the positive effects of exercising may not see a 20- to 40-year drop in your facial youth, but the research is there. Regular physical activity (remember to protect your face from the sun) makes your skin look better and younger. Exercise has been called the low-cost, age-defying beauty regimen that actually works.

If you are enticed by the benefits exercise brings, why not also try the other research-supported, *no* cost, and age-defying beauty regimen, *Skin Sobering*? It takes less effort than exercising, and it gives your skin even more benefits!

POLLUTION

There are a lot of airborne pollutants from automobiles and factories, especially in the city. These pollutants contain nitrogen oxides, ozone, polycyclic hydrocarbons, and volatile organic compounds, all of which contribute to skin problems. Professor Jean Krutmann, director of the Leibniz Research Institute for Environmental Medicine in Germany, found there is a correlation between nitrogen dioxide and age spots (or liver spots).[144] UK cosmetic doctor Mervyn Patterson also found that traffic pollution is a toxic cocktail for the skin and not too different from cigarette smoke damage.[145] Air pollutants, which are very reactive, trigger the skin's inflammatory pathways and activate melanocyte formation. This causes dark spots. In the Eastern world, there's also the concern of yellow dust. This Asian weather phenomenon occurs in the spring and is caused by clouds of desert dust from China. This blows across Japan and Korea, carrying harmful pollutants. To avoid them, people in Seoul wear face masks on days when warnings are issued.

Yes, pollution in the air is harmful to our skin and our body, and that's not only a problem for city dwellers. As reactive as the toxic substances in the cities are, organic and inorganic substances in rural areas are not any less harmful. Pollen, grain dust, airborne particles from pesticides, fertilizers, the burning of stubble, threshing operations, and large-scale use of tractors, combines, and diesel-operated tubes all contribute to tons of pollutants.[146] Our air is not clean. Even if you are lucky enough to live in a low-pollutant region, the wind can bring pollutants from other regions to you. The power of the prevailing wind can move air from China to Japan and Korea, so don't fool yourself that your little bubble of heaven is not going to be affected.

South Korean beauty and product marketers jumped on the scientific bandwagon and twisted the topic so they could sell more products. Now, they claim you need to "protect" your skin by applying products as a shield against the pollutants. This sounds logical, except for the fact that those products weaken and damage the naturally strong protective barrier of the skin and *attract* pollutants rather than deterring them. The Korean beauty regimen of applying 10 products on one's skin is a hot and *heavy* mess of a trend.

Undamaged skin is nature's most resilient defensive mechanism, short of covering yourself in a hazmat suit. You need to keep this barrier intact and strong by protecting it from the sun, making good lifestyle choices, and by nourishing it from within. To say that using skincare products *protects* us from pollutants is illogical in three ways. First, loading chemicals on the skin continues the damage of our natural protective barrier, making it more leaky and susceptible to airborne pollutants. Second, even worse, the texture of these creamy, luxurious substances is like a magnet to pollutants. Think of simple physics. Which surface is going to trap more particles, one that is sticky or one that is sober? Skincare products in fact help to *attract* more pollutants to stick on the skin, hence causing more harm. Third, it is gross to jam this excretory organ that is meant to clear the body's waste.

So, it is correct that we are living among pollutants whether we are in the city or the countryside. The way to defend against pollutants is to have a strong armor. You can wear a mask or head condom to help protect your face. Of course, very few beauty-concerned people want to shield their whole head, even though it would protect the beautiful face they actually want to show the world. Short of a total cover-up (religious reasons aside), your only other option is really to have an intact skin barrier. Your skin is constantly repairing and regenerating, so even if your skin is damaged and leaky, as you remove the assaults—in this context, the biggest culprit is skincare products—your skin will eventually regain its protective strength. It's not too late.

To visualize the skin's natural defensive abilities, think of your nose. Our noses are equipped with natural, pollutant-defending abilities in the form of nasal fluid, hair, and sinuses. Our nose traps pollutants using what nature gave it to protect our lungs. Your extra help would only need to be washing your nostrils daily and rinsing your sinuses with an isotonic solution if needed. You would not use any chemicals to coat your nostrils—or plug them, for God's sake—to prevent pollutants from entering! If your nose needs extra help, wear a mask for physical protection. That is the most you need to do.

Your skin functions the same. It can also handle regular pollution. By lathering chemicals all over your pores daily, you are introducing another pollutant along with its negative effects of clogging, irritation, and inflammation.

SHOCKING FINDING! SKINCARE PRODUCTS ARE THE MOST PROMINENT POLLUTANTS ON THE SKIN

In 2016, a team of researchers from the University of California, San Diego, led by microbiologist Pieter Dorrestein, conducted a study using whole-body mass spectrometry to scan participants' skin.[147,148] Though his goal was to better understand the molecular composition of human skin, the results of his research were unexpected. Dr. Dorrestein remarked, "The largest single source of the molecules found on the skin was not skin cells, nor was it bacteria, fungus or virus. The largest type of 'molecules' were residue from skincare and cleansing products." Without intending to study skincare products at all, Dr. Dorrestein stumbled upon the truth of how toxic these products are for our skin.

Many beauty books and people who sell products try to encourage us to buy products to combat bacteria and pollutants, when in fact the products are the most prominent pollutants!

11

CONFUSION

CONSTANT CELEBRITY ENDORSEMENTS MAKE US TRUST PRODUCTS

THE ILLUSION OF BEAUTY: CELEBRITIES ROCK

A LIFETIME OF BEING MISINFORMED

BUT I SEE YOUR TRUE COLORS SHINING THROUGH

PRECAUTIONARY PRINCIPLE

FROM THE BEAUTY-OBSESSED SCIENTIST

The scientific and medical communities have long been promoting the idea that no makeup and no products are best for the health of your skin. That said, many of us don't want to listen to scientists and doctors nagging us about our health and disregarding our need for glam. Beauty comes first for me! Most people who are concerned about their skin aren't worrying about their skin's *health*. They are thinking about beauty—instant beauty. I wanted to be gorgeous, so the "white coat black art" is not going to be my choice for beauty mentorship.

But skin that is not healthy is also not beautiful. Makeup on a good canvas looks instantly more stunning than makeup on a rag. Make this your incentive if health isn't it.

THE ILLUSION OF BEAUTY: CELEBRITIES ROCK

When it comes to beauty, we pay attention to attractive celebrities and influencers instead of scientists. Those whose professions hinge on beauty or who choose a career in the beauty industry are almost always naturally attractive and were born with good skin. This is different from the medical world, where those who become doctors didn't do it because they were the healthiest, fittest, or even the most health-conscious. Many became doctors because of the prestige, their parents, or a desire to heal.

And the process of becoming a doctor is grueling. So even if physically fit people were as drawn to the medical field as the pretty ones are to the beauty industry and Hollywood, they would find their fitness may fall to the wayside. As the gruesome process of becoming a doctor goes on, fitness and even health often suffers. They have little time to exercise, cook, have relationships, or even to sleep.

What's the takeaway? We listen to doctors about medicine because their advice is logical and scientific, not because they look fit or healthy. On the contrary, we listen to celebrities' messages about beauty purely because they look beautiful, regardless if it's scientific or even logical. Deep down, we might suspect a particular celebrity is unqualified or has a conflict of interest, but it's hard to ignore how great they look. That makes it hard to ignore their message.

Entertainment Tonight Canada was talking about how Jennifer Lopez has beautiful, glowing skin and attributed it to skincare products. First of all, J.Lo was born with it, just like Kristin Bell—I love her skin! Small pores and smooth skin are in their genes. Secondly, J.Lo probably takes extremely good care of herself and has the best makeup artist, stylist, and camera crew. Of course we see her glowing. By the way, what does taking "extremely good care of herself" entail? We've been taught to believe it must be J.Lo's diligent skincare routine, but I bet it has more to do with the active, healthy lifestyle she leads. She may even let her skin be bare whenever she's not facing people. On top of all this, celebrities tend to look good even when their skin is not good or healthy, so don't be shocked if Jenny from the Block is just like us and has bumpy skin when all lights and products are off.

Next is Gwyneth Paltrow, who appeared on a home improvement show *Celebrity IOU* with the Property Brothers. She was demolishing a kitchen and working with hammers in a Canadian tuxedo, so it makes sense that she wasn't wearing much makeup. I was surprised by her wrinkles, crow's feet, and eye puffiness. There's nothing inherently wrong with these things, and if I wasn't researching skin beauty and health, and if she wasn't selling (and presumably using) tons of *goop*, her skin aging signs wouldn't have caught my eye. Her unprepared face seems like a contradiction to the claims made by her products. Gwyneth supposedly leads an exemplary healthy life, but her fortysomething skin is like what my fiftysomething skin was before *Skin Sobering*.

In March 2020, when much of the world was in COVID-19 pandemic lockdown, all the stars were staying home and sending out videos from their homes. Ellen DeGeneres, my favorite talk show lady, revealed her bare face with no makeup. Her skin looked pinkish red, which I guessed was because the daily makeup and skincare products she used for her show were chronically irritating her skin. Pink means inflamed skin. I don't know how many skin chemicals Ellen uses, but the pinkness demonstrates that it's too much.

Ellen also launched a new skin product line called "Kind Science." Oh, Ellen! There's good science, bad science, and fake science. Good science says the skin doesn't need any kind of products. On the day of the "Kind Science" launch, Ellen said she needed a new skincare line because her skin is getting so sensitive.

Ellen doesn't need a new skincare line. She needs *Skin Sobering*.

It can be informative and illuminating when celebrities actually get honest, like when Matilda De Angelis of *The Undoing* shared an unfiltered look at her "face eaten by acne." Her acne is partly due to hormones, but is most likely caused by stress and the products she puts on her skin—an occupational hazard. I would like to chat with Matilda (like the heart-to-heart I had with my stepdaughter, Maggie) to help her (and my favorite Ellen, and J.Lo, Melissa, and Gwyneth!) understand how *Skin Sobering* can rid her biggest acne cause and other skin problems. My Maggie is a beautiful 28-year-old who has practiced *Skin Sobering* for two years. It even got rid of her old acne scars, in addition to giving her great skin that her makeup artist praises.

A camera and good makeup can cover a lot, I know. In one of my Instagram posts, I talked about how great I looked. Who can't look good in photos in this day and age? These posts are not a reflection of how I usually look in person. With special effects, smoothing apps, and 50 or more selfies to "pore" over, you can easily pick out 10 flawless, gorgeous shots to sell whatever you want. This is especially true when it comes to skincare products. That's how beauty influencers do it (I didn't even use any apps, just good lighting). And when I had damaged my skin pretty badly by my 50s, I still looked fine because I would only let people see my best face, one that went through an hour and a half of skillful painting. None of my friends detected that I had bad skin. I bet you that the same goes for these movie stars. We all envy their flawless looks, but make no mistake, their picture-perfect beauty is the result of lots of prep work and talented artists. Underneath all that work, their skin may not be so enviable.

Good-looking people age better as a rule, yet that does not make them qualified to speak about skin care. If you use how attractive a person is to decide whether you will listen to their skin care advice, then the aging dermatologists and the experienced scientists who have dedicated their lives to skin and health will be no match for the Photoshopped influencers. That is the exact phenomenon in our world right now. It is a shame to think we are more willing to listen to those who have beautiful features, beautiful style, and who are beautifully enhanced, than those who are knowledgeable about the science and facts of skin health and beauty.

PRODUCTS AND PROCEDURES CAN DO WONDERS

There are times when skincare products and in-clinic procedures do make a noticeable difference in a person's skin, *if* you have neglected to protect your skin or have indulged in a poor lifestyle for a long time. Skincare commercials often say their lotions and potions will transform your skin in one week. There is some truth to that. True neglect will make your skin dry, rough, and dull. Applying some gooey substance will make any surface look temporarily moist, smooth, and glowy (think again of paint on a canvas). This fleeting enhancement is similar to the effects of the sun. UV rays give you a short-lived glow and tan, but there are layers of harm accumulating underneath what can be seen with the naked eye.

Let's use Melissa McCarthy to illustrate the above point. Why does McCarthy's skin look so much better after she became famous? Watch her in the movie *Bridesmaids*, and then watch her on any recent interviews. In *Bridesmaids*, Melissa's skin was dull, rough, patchy, dry, and uneven. It was perfectly fitting for her character, Megan, who had a bad lifestyle (sorry, Ms. McCarthy, I love your work, just not how your skin looked back then). Now her skin is radiant and smooth. Everybody assumes Melissa's better skin must be the result of using good skincare products. I bet not. I suspect these changes didn't come from skincare products, but from removing layers of accumulated damages from lifestyle choices.

Let's analogize this to teeth whitening. People who didn't look after their skin accumulated years of "stains" not unlike the stains you accumulate on your teeth when you don't take care of them. Whitening the teeth damages both your teeth and gums but it serves a purpose: removing years of discoloration. This results in a whiter smile, a cosmetic benefit you feel is worth some enamel and tissue harm. I bet you when Melissa got famous, some serious "tooth whitening" equivalent was done to her skin to remove her previous skin "stains." She may have used lasers to reduce sun spots, Botox to smooth out lines, chemical peels to get rid of thickened dead skin, makeup to cover up flaws, and skincare products to prime her skin.

I am not advocating these procedures, as there are risks to all of them. Even so, it is only fair to mention there are in-clinic procedures that *can* be effective for treating built-up beauty stains. However, even when they are done by trained and ethical professionals, these options are not without risk and harm of their own.

I suppose some may argue, "Hey, after the tooth stains are gone, you still need to floss and brush with toothpaste daily to maintain dental health and beauty. So, isn't using creams and lotions daily the same maintenance we need for skin?" It is not, for two reasons. First, if you floss and brush daily (with or without toothpaste), you are preventing plaque and gum disease.[149] The *mechanical* action of flossing and brushing plus fluoride is what makes your teeth and gums healthy and keeps them looking good. I use toothpaste during the day because it makes my breath minty fresh—a cosmetic purpose with a social intent. Second, washing your face with water and occasionally pure soap *is* the skin's equivalent of flossing, brushing, and fluoride. Layering products on the skin, an excretory organ, is absolutely redundant. Like the Chinese saying, *drawing feet on snakes* 畫蛇添足 (hua she tian zu), it is as unnecessary and unnatural as can be. As a matter of fact, it's purely wrong.

People doubt *Skin Sobering*, even though the method sells you nothing, takes no time, and simplifies your life. We are so accustomed to reaching for a miracle jar rather than honestly assessing and dealing with the root problem. Even though *Skin Sobering* gives everyone healthier and more beautiful skin, people are still so drawn to gorgeous faces who have no knowledge of product chemistry or skin physiology. Our hardest job will be to oust over 80 years of brilliant soap opera marketing, featuring beautiful stars promising miracle cures for ailments exacerbated *by* these miracle cures.

A LIFETIME OF BEING MISINFORMED

To complicate the beauty advice issue, the beauty arena is almost monopolized by the beauty industry and its spokespeople. Serious scientists don't tend to give skin-deep beauty advice, leaving a big hole for pseudoscience and businesses to take charge.

With so many important world issues, who cares about skin people choose to damage of their own volition? Serious scientists don't want to deal with these shallow problems. It is just skin. But what if our skin is mistreated and misunderstood because of *misinformation*? People have been influenced daily for their entire lives, going back three generations now, with little government regulation or scrutiny. The strongest "education" we've received about our skin is from the beauty industry and beauty doctors (the industry's second-largest sales channel) whose goals are to sell their products.

And beauty schools teach their eager students, future aestheticians, and product salespeople that women have to start a skin care regime at the age they want their skin to look. This beguiling little lie is especially insidious because it lures women into applying products at a young age. And it is an incredibly powerful message—I want to look like I did when I was 20. This is nothing more than the good marketing of a bad idea.

The problems our largest organ faces are not just wrinkles and fine lines. They are eczema and the atopic march in young children, acne and dermatitis in teens, sensitivity and irritation in adults, and inflammation and psoriasis in elders. *This is a public health issue dressed up as skin-deep beauty.* Serious scientists cannot think of it merely as an image issue of insecure or vain women anymore.

Carrie Hammer, a social entrepreneur and luxury fashion consultant, pointed out the obvious at her TEDx Talk: the images presented to us through magazines, videos, and commercials are not real. They are manufactured. These unreal images best serve the beauty industry, not the people. She also reported that we spend more on beauty than education. Together, beauty and fashion are a $1.3 trillion industry—an industry that has been setting unrealistic expectations of beauty, then exploiting and profiting from the insecurities that they helped to create.

She further explained that we have moved beyond mere beauty *illusions*. Now we suffer from *delusion*. When she was a fashion consultant, Hammer worked with 12-year-olds to make them look like perfectly beautiful 30-year-olds on magazine photoshoots. She also designed a magazine cover wherein she visually "replaced" the aged legs of a famous 70-year-old with those from a younger woman using "Frankenstein Photoshop." These unrealistic, digitally enhanced images don't actually exist in real life. They were created through extreme Photoshop, body doubles, and underage girl models—hence the delusion! When we see these expertly, intensely modified images, we feel we are severely inferior. This phenomenon follows us on social media. Even the supposedly most personal of photos might not be real and may have been doctored by plenty of image editing apps. The delusion is no longer the exception.

It's the rule. The altering of these images alters our minds, changes the way we perceive the world, and destroys how we see ourselves.

BUT I SEE YOUR TRUE COLORS SHINING THROUGH

People with naturally great skin are first born with it. That's not their doing. Whether they are going to keep it or destroy it *is* their doing. So, when you see a 20-year-old or an 80-year-old with beautiful skin, don't compare yourself to them. They most likely won the skin lottery. If you must compare, compare them to *themselves*. You can only see whether someone is doing right by their skin by assessing their skin's changes through time. And you have to see them in real life, face-to-face, with bare skin, *and* listen to them describe how their skin feels. That's a level of truth even BFFs may not share, let alone social media influencers. Short of a microscopic assessment, this honesty is the only way you really know if someone has treated their skin well and if it's truly healthy. Any other way just conceals too much of the truth. So, if it is through social media, via advertisement, or under layers of cream, neither you nor *they* are seeing the true color of their skin. It's just all smoke and mirrors, or in *my* case, pride and defiance: "I have to defend my choice, so I can't admit that I've made bad decisions about my face my whole life. I can't be wrong!"

Skin is rarely perceived independently. Rather, it is attached to the whole persona. Bombshell beauties catch our attention regardless of if they have nice skin. The red lips, cat eyes, sculpted brows, highlighted cheeks, charisma, and presence grab our eyes. It is important to remember we are looking at a gorgeous, artistic product of colors and style. Paints and powders obscure actual skin quality or health. If these carefully constructed beauties choose to give credit or call attention to a product, your mind automatically attributes the glamour to the product.

We often confuse done-up skin with great skin, and as a consequence, we mistake what really is responsible for great skin. In contrast, many people with healthy, beautiful skin who choose a look of *au naturel* don't get recognized in the loud, crowded room of delusional bombshell standards, so their true color and method are overlooked too.

LIPS DON'T LIE. EYES TELL THE TRUTH.

Most people believe that skincare products are full of nutrients and have healing powers. We are led to believe the more we use them, the better our skin will be. Let's try to be rational and use our own experience with something very common, like Chapstick, to assess this belief. In this example, we're talking about the nonmedicated kind. The medicated ones are worse.

The more often we apply Chapstick, the dryer our lips eventually feel. This makes us feel like we need more Chapstick. It feels like an addiction. The skin on our lips is thinner, more delicate, more sensitive, and regenerates faster. So, we can feel the effects of a "drug" in this area more immediately and acutely. Lips that feel dry and are in constant "need" of lip balm have become dependent on this "lip crack." The skin on the rest of your body reacts the same way; it's just not as intense. These feelings are signs and symptoms of your skin being mistreated. Your lips don't lie!

And your eyes tell the truth. Due to the temporary effects of skincare products (smoothing, moisturizing, plumping) and the prevalence of image editing, it's hard to see product-related skin damage in photos. However,

> one telltale sign is the eyes. Puffiness, bags, dark circles, or lines are hard to conceal with makeup, and are easy to spot. I know quite a few celebrities personally, and their eyes give away the product damage. These signs are the results of long-term, mild, chronic, and invisible inflammation and irritation—the skin is fighting back. Maybe photo editing apps can erase everything, but these signs are telling in person.

PRECAUTIONARY PRINCIPLE

Now you have been presented with two diametrically opposing beliefs: use skincare products or do *Skin Sobering*. Both claim they will keep your skin healthy and beautiful. One asks you to rely on chemical products that are brilliantly formulated using synthetic compounds or extracted botanicals to care for multiple skin types and conditions. Another asks you to trust nature (before anyone tries to bottle and sell it to you). It asks that you minimize harm—use physical protection to avoid UV damage; live a good lifestyle to avoid accelerated deep layer damage; and use water to avoid chemical damage.

The first, using skincare products, has influenced three generations with marketing claims, celebrity endorsements, medi-spa professionals' recommendations, and friends' testimonies. The second, doing *Skin Sobering*, only has millions of years of history, and is a God-created or nature-evolved method of genuinely natural skin care. There have been lots of *product-to-product* pissing matches between sales representatives—and no matter which product wins, the end result still presents consumers with a product (and both products were probably made by the same company, anyway). Faced with the conundrum of two difficult choices, who should we believe and what should we do? When we are torn between mighty marketing and solid science, why not exercise the precautionary principle?

The precautionary principle is a philosophical and legal approach to methods that lack thorough scientific evidence[150] (which is not the case for *Skin Sobering*, but let's just do this for argument's sake) and have the potential to cause harm. It emphasizes caution, and asks us to pause and reevaluate before diving into something that may be later proven to be detrimental. This principle has become an underlying rationale for environmental protection, health, and food safety.

So, to apply the precautionary principle to skincare products, we must first ask ourselves to consider the worst scenario of each option. Let's apply a timeframe of 30 days. What if using skincare products is indeed wrong and unhealthy, yet we opt to follow that method anyway? Science says our skin will be further damaged; economics says our money will be more depleted; efficiency says our time will be wasted; psychology says our hopes will be crushed, and we will just feel like a fool.

Let's examine the worst case scenario for *Skin Sobering*. If *Skin Sobering* is wrong, then our skin didn't get the chemicals it "needed" for 30 days and got older-looking. But we saved money, time, produced less trash, and our daily routine was simpler for a while.

Hey, if *Skin Sobering* doesn't work, there are lots of miracle creams in stores that ought to be able to fix us, since that is, after all, exactly what they claim. But if *Skin Sobering* works, how much will we—and the world—have gained?

12

HEALTH

...IS HOW WE GET TO BEAUTY

**PAY NOW AND BENEFIT LATER,
OR BENEFIT NOW AND PAY LATER?**

HEALTHY-USER BIAS

COMPLIANCE EFFECT

GROSS WASTE OR NATURAL PROTECTION?

DOES HEALTHY EQUAL BEAUTIFUL?

ATTRACTIVE AUDREY

EXCELLING ERIN

FROM THE BEAUTY-OBSESSED SCIENTIST

PAY NOW AND BENEFIT LATER, OR BENEFIT NOW AND PAY LATER?

The costs of your good habits are in the now, and the benefits are in the future. The costs of your *bad* habits are in the future, and the benefits are in the now (a concept coined by James Clear, author of *Atomic*

Habits). Things like exercising, eating healthier, saving for retirement, and building strong relationships have no immediate reward and take a lot of hard work and willpower. We put time and energy into each thing upfront and enjoy the fruits of our labor later. This is the opposite of instant gratification. With smoking, drugs, sugar, watching Netflix, or scrolling through Instagram, we don't see the damage till much later but we get to enjoy the benefits—the immediate fun and the high—now. This is the model behind the invention of the credit card: why not benefit now and pay later? The reality is, the benefit you get now is fleeting, and the pay you have to fork out later is deep and costly, often with irreversible damage. Tobacco, sugar, and skincare products are examples.

Youth further disguises this "costly future" reality, making it even harder to see the consequences of instant gratification. When our skin is young, we typically won't see many beauty issues yet (except for acne). We feel invincible, even when doing all kinds of bad things. We can bake in the sun, smoke, eat greasy food, have awful sleep, forget to clean our makeup off before bed, or load on skin chemicals. Not much of that damage is visible right away. Sometimes, even when we know we're going to have to pay for something later, "later" seems so far away and feels less pressing.

Youth makes us feel invincible, but as you know, youth is fleeting. The mild signs of dryness and sensitivity and the progression to dullness and fine lines are traps for more skincare products and makeup. This is your skin deteriorating. You are wasting your youth on products with the unnecessary attacks. Once you are no longer seemingly invincible, your skin is vulnerable.

THE ROARING 20S. THE VIBRANT 50S.

You just want to look your best when you are young. Life is short, so you want to experiment, go wild, jazz things up, and be different. YOLO. My stepdaughter played with hair dye a lot. She was purple; she was red; she was silver; and she was black. She wanted her hair to be unique, not just boring brown. But really, she was no different from all the other multicolor heads—all with badly damaged hair and none of them unique (Maggie rolled her eyes so hard when she edited this paragraph, but she didn't change any of it, LOL).

Your youth is your best asset, so you believe your best time is your 20s and 30s. Why look vanilla when you can pump up the volume? Hear me roar! Well, you feel that way because you are young, and you think youth gives you the most advantage and most enjoyment. As a 57-year-old, I've experienced more phases of life, so let me share with you my "wisdom" (and my 85-year-old mom replied, "You haven't seen much yet, kid").

When I was young, my mind was muddy, and I would sweat the big stuff and the trivial things. I had tons of responsibilities: the nonstop demands of my careers and businesses, the total responsibilities of my children's lives; I was learning how to survive my marriages, kinships, and friendships. I had to learn how to be myself and like myself, and I was left with no time or money to really improve or enjoy myself.

My 50s arrived, and time was finally mine. My kids were independent; my parents were still healthy; and I was financially in the best position to enjoy life—and so were my friends! In your 50s, you and your significant other who worked hard on your relationship can now enjoy each other. You and your friends who walked a similar path now have time, health, and money to experience the finer and grander things in life. That's when you want your best self to still be there—feeling good, having amazing places to go, and looking your finest.

If you have been damaging your skin in your 20s, 30s, and 40s (any age, really) with products, you are wasting your skin health and beauty, and your money. Your mild problems, which were likely caused by products, may be masked briefly with more chemical use, but the problems will keep coming back, and getting worse. You have to buy more to fix more, though more products steal more of your future beauty (and money). Then when you hit your 50s, you suddenly see the damage is here to stay, and you blame your age. Well, the truth is you have simply been assaulting your skin long enough that it gave up.

If daily skincare products and regular makeup is how you roll, your face will really pay for it in your 50s and on. You will miss out on having your best looks during the most vibrant time of your life, which is not your roaring 20s.

HEALTHY-USER BIAS

The biggest lure of using products is that the people you see who religiously use skincare products often do look nicer. "How do you explain *that* with your *Skin Sobering* theory, Drs. Tjam and Utsugi?" The answer is something called the "healthy-user bias," which is a form of sample selection bias. Let me walk through a couple of examples to illustrate this.

I heard a guy on the radio the other day discussing a study that showed that those who floss their teeth have better health. The radio guy was pretty smart and pointed out, "Geez, if you bother to floss, you probably bother to exercise, eat well, and do other healthy things." Correct. Flossing is the last frontier; another good thing already healthy people do. This is the healthy-user bias, where it is the positive lifestyle factors and a concern for one's health that actually make these people healthier, not the flossing (in this case actually a good thing, unlike skin chemicals).

As another example, the number of fire trucks sent to combat a fire is positively correlated to the severity of the fire damage. Seems reasonable, but the presence of more fire trucks doesn't cause more severe fire damage. Obviously, sending less fire trucks is not going to lessen the damage! It is a third factor, *the size of the fire*, that is responsible for both.

The bigger the fire, the more trucks are sent. The bigger the fire, the more severe the damage. Fire trucks are not responsible for the damage.

Here's one more. People who take supplements are healthier than the population at large. It seems like supplements are responsible for better health. But when this relationship was examined more closely, it was found that these people's better health had nothing to do with the supplements. Instead, the supplement-takers are better educated and more affluent, so they take a greater-than-average interest in their health. Their education, wealth, and greater health interest are the confounding factors that account for their superior health, not the supplements themselves.

So, why do people who are diligent with using skincare products have nicer-looking skin than those who don't adhere to that routine? Turns out, people who care about their skin also look after their health and have a healthier mindset in general. They are more likely to protect their skin from UV and adjust their lifestyle behaviors to avoid smoking and excessive drinking. These people tend to watch their diet, exercise more, and understand the importance of good sleep.

The fact that they also use skincare products is a reflection of our (mis)belief as a society that skincare products are *good* for us. The real reason for their nicer skin is their greater overall health concerns and their diligence in protecting their skin and adjusting their lifestyle.

Let's examine this further by looking at the counterpart in this comparison: those who don't use skincare products who have *worse* skin. What is the real cause of their worse skin, the lack of product use or something else? Well, I'm quite certain that many who do nothing to their skin, who choose no skincare products, did not do so because of a solid knowledge of *Skin Sobering*. Chances are, people in this group most likely just don't bother much with their looks. They may not even protect their face from the sun or adjust their lifestyle indulgences. It just isn't as important to them.

When you have two "wrongs" like failing to protect your skin and having bad lifestyle habits, one "right" in the form of avoiding skincare products isn't going to help as much as you might have hoped. Conversely, when you have two "rights" like protecting your skin and living a healthy life, one "wrong" in slathering on chemicals isn't going to rear its ugly head as soon as it should.

There is another layer to the healthy-user bias with respect to skin appearance and skin care. Diligent skincare product users are also likely to fuss a lot over their looks—their hair, clothes, makeup, and overall "put-togetherness." This creates a halo effect because when we see people who are more put together, we automatically perceive that they look better as well. We associate good-looking people with good-looking everything, including skin. So, skincare users get two unearned credits with regard to their skin. First, their better skin is misattributed to the use of skincare products when the real heroes were protecting skin and adjusting habits. Second, their skin is perceived as better than it is just because they are perceived as more attractive.

COMPLIANCE EFFECT

What perhaps is as significant as heathy-user bias in explaining why skincare product users may look better is the compliance (or adherer) effect.[151] Medically, this refers to a phenomenon where people who are compliant with a treatment may differ from those who don't comply. The difference is so great that it could affect the outcome being measured.

Studies show that people who comply with an intervention are different and healthier than people who don't, regardless of whether the intervention is beneficial or not. [152] Healthy-user bias and compliance effect can make even a harmful effect appear as if it is helpful just because the users are healthier to start with and will follow through with things. So, are skincare products giving these people better skin, or did these people start off with healthier habits and are compliant with life's healthy ways? Unfortunately, it is clear these diligent people just listened to the wrong skin care messages and grew up believing in marketing instead of science.

GROSS WASTE OR NATURAL PROTECTION?

We don't like the feeling of our own oil, but we welcome the oils in manufactured creams and lotions. We think of our own secretions as gross, so we strip them all off only to quickly apply the purchased chemicals. Can you see how much our feelings are commercially conditioned?

Skincare and cosmetic companies spend billions of dollars on R&D to try to create products that mimic our bodily substances. Meanwhile, we obsessively wash our own miracle secretions away, disrupting and destroying the body's natural functions only to replace them with an inferior chemical perpetrator, or grosser—animal urine, vomit, and semen.

Yes, I said *semen*.

You can Google "animal products used in cosmetic creams and lotions" if you're feeling brave.

We are made to think of our sebum as yucky, oily gunk that we can't wait to wash completely off. To illustrate this ingrained misconception, let's use our saliva and nasal fluid as contrasts. Liquid inside your nose is gross, spit is gross—yes, if you touch someone else's (unless you are in love with them, in which case their saliva is heaven's dew and you yearn to negotiate a French exchange). Nasal fluid and saliva are however necessary and supposed to be where they are produced: inside your nose and mouth. Imagine if you completely stripped your nose and mouth dry. Without any wetness in these two cavities, they would feel extremely uncomfortable and would not function properly. A dry mouth and a dry nose is a torturous experience. We recognize that feeling and are not dumb enough to create it deliberately. We also know better than to ever attempt to smear chemical "moisturizers" in our nose or mouth to replenish the natural moisture that *we just stripped away.*

The gravely misunderstood feelings of dryness, sensitivity, itchiness, and redness are also torture, but we have accepted them as normal feelings of the skin. Decades of commercials have conditioned us to expect that "squeaky clean" feeling, which also gives us dry and sensitive skin. What do they tell us we need for dry, sensitive skin?

Their products.

Sensitive skin is a warning that the skin's essential, natural protectors are gone. Our body needs its natural substances where they are produced to keep our body functioning well even though scientifically they are called "bodily wastes." Tears, saliva, nasal fluids, ear wax, vaginal discharge, sweat, and sebum all fall into this category. We should not strip all of these substances off. We do need to wash the dirty and oxidized secretions off twice a day with lukewarm water. We need wetness inside our nostrils and eyes; we need saliva in our mouth; and we need sweat and oil on our skin to be healthy. Who taught us to hate our natural secretions?

If you worry about cleanliness, you are probably clean. With most product-dependent people, they are likely overcleaning rather than undercleaning. Remember, the Centers for Disease Control and Prevention (CDC) states its goal for hygiene practice is *to provide adequate protection from transmission of infecting agents while minimizing the risk for changing the ecology and health of the skin.*

Change your perspective of cleanliness to the standard of *health and science* rather than *claims and marketing.* This will save your skin. Stripping your skin clean with products is unhygienic! Killing off all your bacteria is unhealthy! It is excessive and damaging to your skin! Water is the only agent that doesn't change the ecology and health of our skin. That's what good doctors have been telling the beauty-conscious for ages but *honest words prick the ears* 忠言逆耳 (zhong yan ni er)—the truth hurts. But ignorance kills.

DOES HEALTHY EQUAL BEAUTIFUL?

Skin Sobering is proven by science and backed by clinical data: it makes skin more beautiful. It is not just to reduce skin sensitivity or get rid of diseases. Many books written by great doctors don't catch on to this distinction. The mother of all reasons for skincare, for most people, is to make their skin beautiful, regardless of health. Many don't mind the unhealthy measures they have to take—even if they do understand they are harming their skin with products.

Worse? Some people mistake this temporary look or feel *for having healthy skin*.

The good doctors who use a health- and disease-oriented approach to discourage product use were *playing the zither to the cows* 對牛彈琴 (dui niu tan qin)—sending a good message to the wrong audience. The users won't listen. The beauty-obsessed want their skin to be youthful, smooth, radiant, clear, luminous, glowing, dewy—essentially near perfection. They are *picking bone out of an egg* 雞蛋裡挑骨頭 (ji dan li tiao gu tou)—a condition that doesn't exist. It is excessively demanding, worse than nitpicking. They don't just want their skin to be flawless; they want it "pore-less." Chasing rainbows is why people seek out all this skincare stuff and buy into all this shit.

All cultures have ways of torturing their people in the name of beauty. Eastern women bleach their skin to look fair, eat tapeworms to stay thin, bind their feet to a *3-inch lotus* 三寸金蓮 (san cun jin lian)—to seem dainty, and elongate their necks with metal coils to look attractive. Don't roll your eyes at these foolish Easterners. Western women bake in the sun to get color, take drugs to stay thin, binge and puke to lose weight, surgically remove their ribs for a smaller waistline, wear high heels for longer legs, bind their teeth with wire for a greater smile, and inject plastic in their cheeks, lips, and boobs to look firm. You name a culture and I guarantee that culture has its own method of beauty-driven torments.

Societies have globalized, and the East and the West are copying each other's torture games. I began thinking about beauty as young as age 6. I rubbed on talcum powder to look white, didn't rinse out conditioner in order to have more silky hair, forced myself to eat beef to get rid of freckles (I hated beef. It was my mom's fib to get me to eat beef—she meant well). I am older and I got smarter, so I won't trade health for beauty anymore. And isn't it marvelous that *Skin Sobering* is all about getting your skin more beautiful with the side benefit of health?

I have always dug around to learn how to be more beautiful. It's a tiring pursuit, but it's very satisfying when you uncover real answers. In spite of all the things we do to enhance our beauty, if our skin has problems, we'll end up *doubling our efforts and halving our results* 事倍功半 (shi bei gong ban). The opposite is even more relevant. When our bare skin is healthy and beautiful, we require only half the effort to see double the results.

So, this book is not seeking to turn you into a granola, an *au naturel* who never touches makeup, nor is it to make you discard your meticulously curated style. It is to show you how to restart your skin and get rid of its problems so you have a wonderful, healthy base to work your enhancement magic—with *half the effort* 事半功倍 (shi ban gong bei). That's effortless beauty.

HAIR DRYER AND IRON

There are many things we do to make ourselves look prettier, and we are quite aware of their costs and benefits. Let's talk about hair again. We blow dry and flat iron our hair to make the strands momentarily smoother, shinier, curlier, or straighter. We know heat can give us that effect, but we also know heat can damage our hair. So, we only use heat when we need to look good for that day. We don't use heat to curl or straighten before we go to sleep, nor do we do it frequently in the hope that the smoothness, curls, or shine will become permanent. We know this visual benefit is short-lived. As soon as our hair gets wet, the cuticles lose that heat-induced effect.

Products for the skin are like heat for the hair. They are not nutritious treatments capable of making your skin smooth and radiant for good. They are temporary fixes with definite, lasting damage. At least Dyson is honest about their hair irons, "Designed for enhanced styling, with half the damage." If skincare products carried more truthful messages like flat irons and cigarette warning labels do, the responsibility for using skin chemicals would at least truly be on us.

If you want your hair to stay shiny and smooth by ironing it all the time, you may have shiny-looking hair, but before too long, you won't have much hair left to shine. In a similar fashion, use skin chemicals like you would a hair iron, indulging only when you want their temporary effects. Don't mistake either of them as nourishment or care.

OCCUPATIONAL HAZARD

People who need to wear makeup every day for television are in a tough situation. Realistically, they probably cannot avoid being painted by products. If your job is to face the world every day under lights and cameras and be seen by millions of people, well, that is a level of stress most of us don't have. The entertainment world requires its participants to glam up. There's little we can do to change that, not unless the industry drops this demand (if only barefaced ambassador Alicia Keys could win this war). Dedicated doctors with bad health, elite athletes with joint immobility, chefs with poor eating habits—these are such ironic occupational hazards, just like good-looking stars who wreck their skin to temporarily look better for their audiences.

For those of you who give us wonderful entertainment at the daily expense of your natural skin, we hope you have afternoons off, evenings off, weekends off, and some long holidays where you are able to allow your skin to metabolize and regenerate without an onslaught of daily chemical disruptions. Just use water and don't put anything on your face on those days, evenings, and nights. As long as you give your skin a chance to sober up, it will have a chance to recover. When there comes a day (or you create that day), where you begin to not use them for 30 days, you will start to be free, from both chemicals and your skin issues.

NATURAL MAKEUP

An up-and-coming Chinese beauty YouTuber with over 500K subscribers advocates using a simple method to achieve a "quiet" and "light" no-makeup look. I'm not against makeup, but I do question the reasons people use it. If it is to achieve a quite natural look, why not improve your skin condition so you can have that truly natural glow?

What products were used to manufacture the trendy "no-makeup" look? I won't include this YouTuber's list because it is over 20 items long! It included products like primer, correctors, concealers, multiple foundations, mascaras, powders, shadows, blushes, lip balm, and lipstick, all to achieve a product-free look.

If it takes over 20 products to create a product-free look, imagine how many it takes to get done up for Oscar night! Like many influencers, that same YouTuber very likely showed us *that* many products because she gets paid for each product mentioned. She herself also uses that many products because when we see her real, bare skin, it is gray, dull, and blemished by acne and acne scars—a clear sign of product damage. Even if she doesn't usually use 20 or more products for that "natural" look, she is teaching and advertising this 20-product method to half a million people. These people trust what she has to say enough that they've subscribed to her social channel. She might even believe in what she's selling, too, and she may have no idea why her bare skin is struggling. She has convinced half a million followers to believe that more products equals more beauty, even though her own bare skin reveals the opposite situation.

This whole trend of "no-makeup" makeup clearly doesn't mean using less makeup. It just means you use different products with different techniques. So much work for subtlety! When your skin recovers, it is beautiful without makeup. When your skin gets healthy, your no-makeup look truly won't need makeup.

We know makeup is a must if we want our lips cherry red and our eyelids baby blue. Unfortunately, there's no other way. Makeup adds color, covers color, brightens color, and changes color, so makeup is a must for achieving these unnatural, lovely looks.

Conversely, skincare products are *not* a must. The advertised purpose of skin chemicals is to give us healthier and more beautiful skin, but using them actually destroys *exactly* that. Skin care companies' current claim is not that different than if tobacco companies were to rave that cigarettes can cure lung cancer or if the sugar industry began to praise sugar for helping weight loss. Even those two powerful giants couldn't bend the truth like that. But the skin care industry is doing just that. Science and clinical data have shown that skincare products *create* damage and *speed up* aging, yet their advertisements are implying these products prevent skin damage and slow down aging.

Skincare products do *not* serve their purpose of making your skin healthier.

ATTRACTIVE AUDREY

What aspects of our face make us attractive and beautiful? On his YouTube channel, Dr. Gavin Chan from the Victorian Cosmetic Institute in Australia asked why Jane Fonda looks so young even though she is in her 80s. Is it because of plastic surgeries and careful treatments? There's much more to it. Joan Rivers had lots of surgeries and treatments, as have many other women, but none of their results compare to Fonda's. Good skin or not, they looked overdone and not attractive.

Many women who want to look beautiful are obsessed with the *surface* of their face—the frown lines, the lip lines, the crow's feet, the folds, and the wrinkles. "These don't matter that much and don't take away from one's good looks," explained Dr. Chan. What really determines attractiveness are the big things (we know inner beauty is the biggest one).

Attractiveness is not determined on a plane; it has more than two dimensions. Unfortunately, the two-dimension view is what people gravitate toward. They look in a mirror and scrutinize an area. With that mindset, all they find are lines, folds, and discoloration. Predictably, those are problems they want to fix. In spite of this two-dimensional focus, attractiveness is instead truly judged by our eyes in a three-dimensional way, taking our face's shape, contour, and proportions into account. If you are saggy and shapeless, that draws the eyes much more than crow's feet and laugh lines. So, someone with a good bone structure, a nice jawline, high cheeks, and especially a good physique will look attractive whether there are lines on their face or not. These three-dimensional features determine our beauty and physical appeal much more than lines and color.

Dr. Chan further explained that Jane Fonda was very attractive as a young girl. That's her key advantage (again, the genetic lottery), as good-looking people age better as a rule. However, if you don't feel you won the genetic lottery, the following factors are even more important. As we get older our face becomes more and more disproportionate, with facial sagging and volume loss. Fonda has kept up her fitness (for the uninitiated, she pioneered VHS workout tapes), and she has led a very healthy lifestyle. Exercise has been shown to slow aging at a cellular level, and there's no doubt this is what happened with Jane Fonda. She protects her skin from the sun, and she eats a healthy diet of fresh food, minimal red meat, and not too many carbs. She doesn't smoke, doesn't overindulge in alcohol, and she meditates.

In an interview with *Healthy Living Magazine*,[153] she said, "Trying to be intentional about how we live, staying interested, staying curious, paying attention to young people, cultivating young friends, these kinds of things are, I think, important to staying youthful." It's not that Jane Fonda looks 40 or 50, it is that she looks attractive at her age that makes her so appealing.

I love Ms. Fonda's work so much, so it pains me to point out her skin health issues here (I'm sorry, Jane). However, this further proves Dr. Chan's point that the two-dimensional plane doesn't determine attractiveness. Looking at untouched photos of Jane Fonda, we see that her skin is crinkly, dry, and wrinkly (look up "Jane Fonda arrested"—she's wearing a red coat). Her skin looks so different in these photos than in her prepared images.

Yes, she is in her 80s and we should never expect young skin from her. My mom is 85 and she's not stylish and attractive like a movie star, but her skin is smooth, hydrated, and supple. My mom doesn't use skin products, and she's had no professional help with her style—just me, trying, but she listens to her younger, 75-year-old friends more than me.

Jane Fonda is blessed with many beautiful traits and has invested a great deal into her looks. In the attractiveness department, Fonda has done almost everything right! Her fitness, her style, her hair, her makeup, and her grace are all on point. But looking solely at her skin? It has taken some beatings, as revealed in her untouched images. I can make an educated guess that the only thing she has done wrong is a lifetime of using skincare products she thought were good for her skin health but instead destroyed it.

No different than most women, I bet Jane Fonda trusts skincare products. Why else would her skin be the only thing that looks older than the rest of her? If she didn't use so many products in her lifetime, her skin would currently match the rest of her. Unfortunately, she didn't know, and she has been living in blissful ignorance like most beauty-conscious people.

You can start *Skin Sobering* in your 80s. It is not too late. My mom started at 82, and now her skin looks like it did in her 60s. Yours can too, Ms. Fonda.

Speaking of grace, elegance, and the big things that define attractiveness, let us return to the iconic Audrey Hepburn. Ms. Hepburn is the personification of beauty and class. Not only did she grace the stages of film and theater, but her glamor extended into real life as well. She is one of Hollywood's greatest fashion and style icons and represented a perfect mixture of sensitivity, strength, and willpower. Of all her public accolades, the best praise came from her friends. They said they never saw her angry, jealous, selfish, temperamental, or cranky. She was always kind and thoughtful, and she carried a smile and a kind word for everybody. She sounds like she was a princess out of a fairy tale.

Unfortunately, this princess also smoked a lot, drank, and suffered from anemia. Audrey Hepburn died far too young. Cancer took her at the age of 63.

When someone is as free and passionate as Audrey Hepburn, whether they have beautiful skin or not matters nil. This skin-deep book is really shallow when you reflect on the true meaning of beauty and attractiveness. Hepburn often quoted American humorist Sam Levenson when she recited, "For beautiful eyes, look for the good in others; for attractive lips, speak words of kindness; and for poise, walk with the knowledge that you are never alone."

When we examine examples like Jane Fonda and Audrey Hepburn, it is clear their style, fitness, grace, and sensibility are what make them beautiful, and their actual skin doesn't matter that much. So, spend your time and money on physical health, mental agility, and emotional maturity. Work on self-awareness, tolerance of others, and broaden your perspective. Improving these things will make you much more beautiful than the lines on your face. Your actual skin, now that you know what makes it beautiful and healthy, should require the least of your attention.

EXCELLING ERIN

My name Yuet 越 in Chinese means "to excel and overcome—超越." My Ba had high expectations of me. In turbulent times, to survive you must overcome.

Friends who have known me for a long time say that I actually look quite young for my age. So they say whatever skin care routine I did before must have worked. Well, I don't think it's my previous skin care routine that saved my skin. It was my lifestyle routine. Even though I have damaged my skin with products for years, I have also done many things right. I don't like sweets; I can't stand dairy; I eat a lot of vegetables; I do not prefer roasted, grilled, or barbecued foods; I drink a ton of water; I don't drink alcohol; I've never smoked; I avoid the sun on my face; and I exercise regularly. The skin conditions I've never had to complain about are elasticity, collagen, fullness, and volume. Those otherwise common beauty complaints are the things that were helped by my good lifestyle. That, alongside my three-dimensional features, makes me look young.

Remember, before *Skin Sobering*, I suffered from 22 skin problems. These were all issues aggravated *by products* that I was trying to correct *with products*. Of course, the issues never got better but they could be covered up with skincare and makeup products. Every time the products were off, my face no longer looked young.

Once, I flew to China with my friend Brenda Halloran, the mayor of Waterloo. I was wearing a full face of skillfully applied natural makeup when we boarded the plane. After our 15-hour flight, the makeup was melted. Brenda saw me as we were exiting the flight and exclaimed, "Geez, what happened to your face?" My very kind, polite friend was so shocked by my real skin that she lost her poise, LOL.

My skin issues only got better after I stopped using products. As I've mentioned before, *Skin Sobering* solved 20 of the 22 problems I had with my skin. My youthful looks then were a result of living a healthy lifestyle and applying great makeup techniques. My problems then were a result of skincare products. The following graphic is how I summarize my beauty practice and beauty results.

Since I started *Skin Sobering*, I've made even more health changes to further excel in the lifestyle arena. I can do that—surprise!—because I have more time and money from not wasting them on product routines and products. Besides what I've already been doing, I now eat one meal a day consisting of mostly plants, and I fast for 48 hours once a

BEFORE

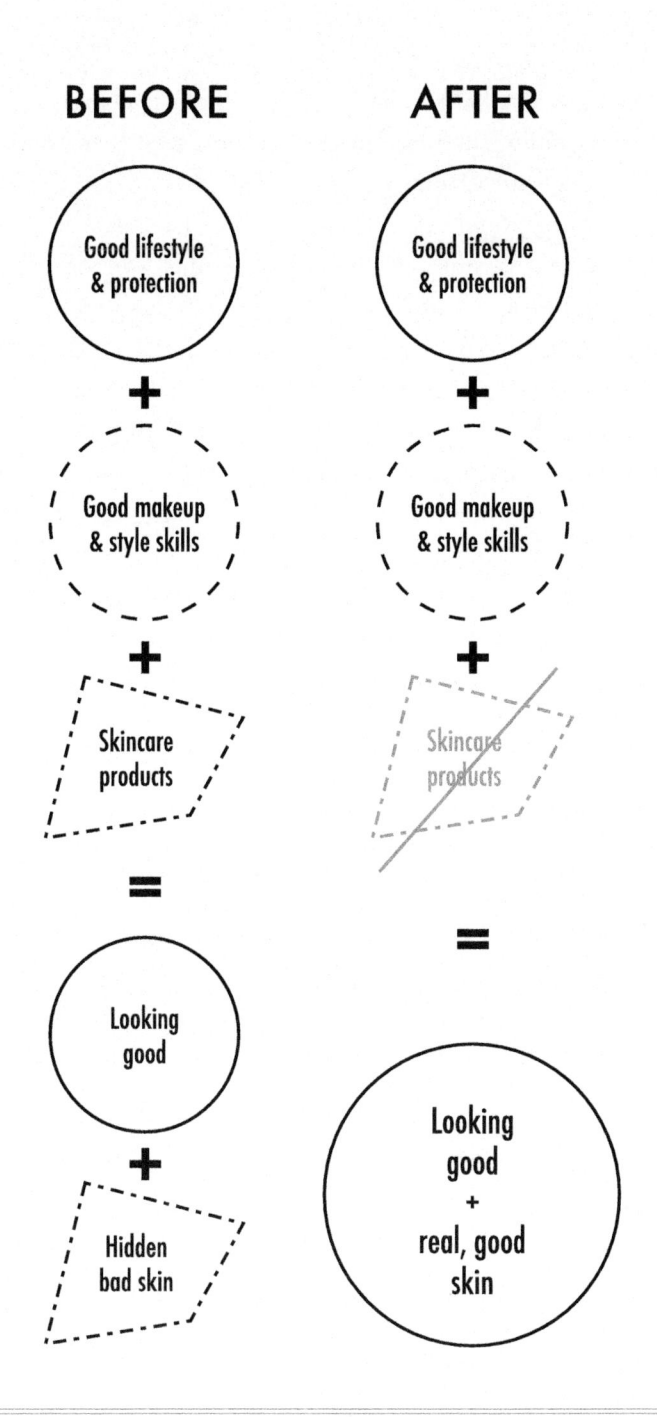

(Good lifestyle & protection)

+

(Good makeup & style skills)

+

[Skincare products]

=

(Looking good)

+

[Hidden bad skin]

AFTER

(Good lifestyle & protection)

+

(Good makeup & style skills)

+

[~~Skincare products~~]

=

(Looking good
+
real, good skin)

HEALTH · 239

week. I sweat each day through simple, full-body exercises, along with yoga, cycling, skiing, and housework. I have also started playing pickleball every day since January 2022, so the 48-hour fasting frequency has been reduced. Some would question how I know that it's not my lifestyle changes that improved my skin instead of *Skin Sobering*. I'm not a lab rat nor a research subject, so I'm not going to run a study on myself. If I'm looking better, I'm keeping all the good changes, especially when they save me time and money and are scientifically sound. When you start one good change, don't be surprised when other good changes follow, including mental agility and emotional maturity.

Don't try to use products to look young. Trying to drop a decade from your face will require a lot of resources and will result in disappointment, frustration, and regret. Reallocate the time and energy you spend trying to look young, and spend it instead on living well and being happy.

13

CHANGE

DROP THE MARKETING NONSENSE AND ADOPT NEW BEHAVIORS BASED ON SCIENCE

WITHDRAWAL

PAMPERING

NOISES

KIM KARDASHIAN OR ROSA PARKS

FROM THE BEAUTY-OBSESSED SCIENTIST

When we are young, inexperienced, and regenerative, we may experiment with many bad things, and we can probably get away with them. Youth and its restorative powers will likely correct minor harms, like a bad hangover, an upset stomach, or an all-nighter. The difficulty is changing a *habit*—a behavior that is already a routine and that we repeat regularly. That's why people who check their phone obsessively and claim they will reduce use can't; why people who sleep in late and mean to stop fail; why those who are in bad relationships and want to change are unable to; and it is why people who use skincare products daily and want to quit have such a hard time.

Changing a habit requires psychological and physiological preparedness. The Stages of Change Model demonstrates that to make a change, one must go through a cyclical process of precontemplation, contemplation, preparation, action, and maintenance.[154] In other words, changing takes willpower and discipline.

By now, we have all heard that refined sugars and simple carbohydrates are not good for us. So why aren't people quitting them? The first reason is that many people still don't believe these substances are *really* a problem. They are still fooled by the conventional wisdom of the '80s. Back then, the predominant marketing message was that fat is bad and sugar is fine. They also can't get through the quitting phase to arrive at the beneficial place. Sugar tastes too good, so people don't want to give it up—this is besides the fact that they are already addicted to it.

Pediatric endocrinologist Dr. Robert Lustig's *Sugar: The Bitter Truth* has been viewed 13 million times on YouTube.[155] Lustig is the lucky one, unlike his predecessor Dr. John Yudkin. Yudkin sounded the alarm on sugar back in 1972 in a book called *Pure, White, and Deadly*. After its release, Yudkin's career and reputation were destroyed because prominent nutritionists—alongside the food industry itself—shut him and his message down. Yudkin died a disappointed man and a forgotten scientist. North Americans ignored his findings, and death by obesity, heart disease, and diabetes rose exponentially.

In previous chapters, Dr. Utsugi and I have drawn a comparison between skincare products and sugar. In light of Drs. Yudkin and Lustig's stories, we fear these two product categories may have shockingly similar outcomes. Are Dr. Utsugi and I going to be dragged like Yudkin, our reputations and careers destroyed by prominent dermatologists and beauty brands while millions more people go on to suffer from skin diseases? Or are we going to be lucky like Lustig and find that millions are prepared to change because of *Skin Sobering*'s message? Will our path be smooth or full of obstacles? You can help us shape it.

Quitting a habit or changing any behavior is not an easy process. More than 90% of people will not succeed the first time they try to quit smoking.[156] With skincare products, there's an added difficulty. By now, most people already have a proper understanding of tobacco, processed foods, and even social media. They understand that these things are not good for them, and they are slowly finding ways to make changes. This is what's known as the preparation and action stage. Unfortunately, the skincare and cosmetic industry is too brilliant. We are not even at the stage of *being aware* of what skin chemicals do to our skin. So, we are in a *pre*-precontemplation phase. Just like the flat Earth beliefs of the 16th century, "healthy" smoking in the 1940s, baby formula battles of the 1960s, rampant episiotomies in the 1970s, and ballooning sugar consumption of the 1980s, our current understanding of skin chemicals is in its ignorant, ancient times. We still use them on newborns! Imagine how far we are from actually completing the Stages of Change Model and terminating skincare product use.

WITHDRAWAL

We hope this book has armed you with enough facts to believe that skin needs many things to be healthy and beautiful, but it does not need or want chemicals. With this new belief comes action, and the action of quitting anything is never easy. You may encounter many hurdles, and the first one will be the uncomfortable but necessary withdrawal reaction.

A withdrawal reaction (also referred to as the Herxheimer reaction) means you will feel worse before you feel better. The withdrawal effect is the combination of physical and mental issues that you experience after you stop using or reduce the use of a substance. A substance with high addictiveness may result in a person experiencing anything from discomfort to vomiting. Missing one's routine morning coffee, for instance, might result in fatigue, headaches, and irritability. Withdrawal symptoms vary depending on the type of substance that was being used or abused.

When we use a substance regularly for a long time, our body will build a tolerance and dependence on that substance. Tolerance means it takes a larger amount of the substance to achieve the same effects that were initially experienced, while dependence means your body needs that substance to avoid experiencing withdrawal reactions. Withdrawal symptoms are usually the opposite of the effects of the substance. For example, alcohol is a depressant, so if a regular, moderate user suddenly stops consuming alcohol, they might experience symptoms of overstimulation, such as anxiety or restlessness.

In the case of *Skin Sobering*, your skin may get worse before it gets better. After long-term use of chemicals, skin builds up tolerance. It starts to need more and more skincare products to mask the initial problems. However, if you stop using the products, your skin may feel dry, oily, itchy, or flaky—whatever your initial problem was. These are problems that products caused and are the withdrawal symptoms of dependency on these products.

So, when you first begin *Skin Sobering*—whether you quit cold turkey or go about it gradually—your skin may feel bad. Hang in there. You are still just grappling with the newfound truth that cleansers lead to more oil, and moisturizers cause dryness, and now you have to deal with quitting them and feeling bad without them. That is hard to take. Similar to quitting any substance that you've been dependent on, you will need to go through a cleansing process, and it may have some ugly stages. The ugly is necessary to get rid of the dependency and the damage that skincare products have caused your skin. Give it 30 days. The withdrawal period for skin chemicals is much shorter than it is for alcohol, and you will benefit just as much.

MAKING THE CHANGE EASIER

Sustaining a new habit and making it a lifelong practice requires that we find encouragement and enjoyment in the process. A belief you will eventually like the end benefits may not be enough to get you there. If you can find perks in the process of creating a new habit, your chance of success will be greater.

For the last two years, I've been successfully fasting 48 hours once a week, and I eat only one meal a day otherwise. This is not just because of the end benefits of autophagy, anti-inflammation, cell renewal, and weight control. I also enjoy not cooking two extra meals every day. It's nice to not be constantly washing dishes. I love the additional time I've gained to read, write, work, socialize, exercise, and play. I like the money I save on groceries. I look forward to the amazing flavors and satiety I'm guaranteed to have each time I eat. There's no more "What should I eat?" quandary. All good foods taste amazing when your gastrointestinal system is working well! The benefits of better health and being able to eat what I love without guilt make fasting a great habit to have. There's nothing better than loving the process *and* the results.

Could *Skin Sobering* be a new habit where you can love the process and the results? Think of these extra perks: time saved from not using skincare products; counter space recovered from bottles and jars; travel packing made easier; money recuperated; the environment is better preserved; and all the benefits that accompany a simpler, less stressful life. As for the big prize at the end? As a result of removing irritation, invasion, disruption, and inflammation from this vitally important excretory organ, your skin will be healthier and more beautiful.

PAMPERING

To many, products represent pampering. To give up products means to give up pampering. That's hard.

It is so nice to pamper myself once in a while. I fuss over my looks when I have an important event, when I'm going to meet old friends I haven't seen in a long time, and when I want to be extra sweet to my Bruce. Doing all this on a daily basis would be too tiring, and it would lose its magical effect. Also, I would feel narcissistic and indulgent.

I have a lot of other things to do each day, and I want to do them. I love to cook; I want to ferment foods and drinks; I need to play; I have to take care of my business; I long to see my friends and chat about home improvements, sports vacations, ways to break our husbands of their nasty habits, and debunking new beauty myths; and I must write. I also have endless things to chat about with my mom, like her grandkids, chickens, ducks, fish, cats, veggies, swimming, church, good and nasty friends, relatives, her daily driving adventures through annoying road construction, her health, and her emotions. A lot of stories are packed into her 85 years.

My husband and I love house parties and cooking up big feasts. He likes tasting many types of scotch, tequila, and wines, and since I won't touch these yucky-tasting liquids (I've tried) with a 10-foot pole, I am the perfect designated driver. We sing way past sociable hours (karaoke mostly, unless our musical sons and relatives are with us and jamming with real instruments), all the while ensuring food is not in short supply. I love all of the above, and the requests from our six grown kids for family dinners. It used to be that we had to butter them up to make them stay for a meal. Now, we are somehow cool parents (or free food) and our kids, their significant others, and their friends all want to come over often. It is a priceless feeling that they now want to be with us and have long chats with us after those trying teen years. Still, cooking meals for 16-plus people is no picnic. So, I don't have time to pamper myself regularly, and I don't want to. It would make the pampering feel ordinary, and most of the desired effects would be gone or diluted.

On those special occasions when I do choose to pamper myself, I will take a long shower and shave. I will pluck, check every pore on my face, suck in here, perk up there, and strike the best pose. I will spend hours looking through my wardrobe, pairing up outfits and shoes and taking selfies—or I'll make Bruce take the shot from a better angle. I will put on makeup if I am going out, and I will take even more selfies, this time close-up. I feel stylish, attractive, and confident. When the event is over, I can't wait to remove everything—my tight bra, high-waisted panties, five-inch stilettos, and my whole face. I thank the heavens above for an end to this ordeal, and I feel grateful that I don't have to do this again for at least another month or two.

Pampering has not only become deeply linked with products, but it is also synonymous with self-care and "me time." That makes it hard for us to separate products from pampering. I'm not being sanctimonious here, but there are lots of other activities you can do without clogging your excretory organ. You want touchy-feely? Get a body massage. You want quick and easy? Take a foot bath. You want hot and steamy? Spring for a sauna or steam shower. And if you want quiet and private, read a lusty novel; for tasty and satisfying, cook up a feast; for wet and sunny, go to the beach! If you want to get sweaty and get your adrenaline pumping, go for a run, ride a bike, hike, or ski—whatever is available in your area!

For some, going to a spa means mother-daughter bonding time or a chance to connect with girlfriends. So, no facials would mean less of this precious time together! Thankfully, this is not the case. There are lots of other activities! Plan a fun meal together—I mean, get a good recipe, actually go grocery shopping together, and cook together. Do yoga, bike to a little country town, sign up for weekly lessons to learn a fun activity like skiing or painting. Volunteer at a charity together, go to a concert, or have a book-finding day—actually go to a bookstore together, find something you and your friends like, and follow up with a book club. Visit your parents or grandparents. Organize a tidying-up party—go to each other's closets, try on each other's clothes, and declutter each other's excess. These all don't involve spas or skincare products, and are just as much fun, or more.

Skincare products are not so bad that they will give you cancer. At least, we hope they won't. We still don't know how all these chemicals accumulate in our body and how we respond to their buildup at the cellular level from contact, inhalation, or ingestion. For now we know skincare products are just not good for our skin, and chemicals are not needed by our body. Pamper yourself in hundreds of other ways. Your skin deserves to be left alone to do its own natural pampering.

NOISES

"Visibly smoother, brighter skin in just 24 hours."
—No-name model, for Olay

"How do you get skin happy 24/7?...You'll look like this [me] and feel like this [my great life]."
—Jennifer Aniston, for Aveeno

"For smoother skin in one day, younger skin in one week..."
—Jennifer Garner, for Neutrogena

"Skincare that boosts your natural rosy tone. It's natural, it just comes from the inside."
—Jane Fonda, for L'Oréal

"Get brighter eyes in a blink."
—Helen Mirren, for L'Oréal

"Love, beauty, and planet. Vegan and cruelty-free. Bottles made from 100% recycled material."
—Ellen DeGeneres, promoting environmentally friendly and humane products

"Something that's clean, sustainable, inclusive..."
—Victoria Beckham, pitch of her products

There are countless, 30-second promotional noises trying to sell these products to us, and there are even more in-depth "interviews" aiming to alter our perspective. In advertising, it is now a common practice to write marketing pieces that look so similar to *actual health articles* that most consumers cannot tell the difference. Consumers believe they're reading the results of something far more unbiased than it actually is, and they buy products as a result.

How easy is it to believe in skincare products when so many celebrities, talk show hosts, aestheticians, cosmetic MDs, friends, and even our family all tell us that products make us beautiful? Then there's the psychological phenomenon of the *mere exposure effect*. One of these ads are in my face every couple of minutes. I couldn't watch TV or YouTube without some skincare magic talk creeping into my brain.

Speaking of magic, the brilliant marketers of L'Oréal have once again pounced, making another claim for their hyaluronic acid-infused conditioner: "It's not magic, it's science." Everyone is now jumping on the science bandwagon. Companies are dropping their *magical* and *miracle* taglines, replacing them with promises of (fake) science. Brilliant.

It's so easy to believe in these products when they are endorsed by beautiful people, come in lovely bottles, have pretty smells, attractive packaging, exotic ingredients, do-good-to-the-earth messages, and make such enticing promises. This is all powered by *Mad Men*-level marketing. If the first jar they sold us was disappointing, it's not hard to get a second one, something else new, shiny, and gorgeous, made of myths and hope.

Skin chemical commercials like to claim the impossible. They say these products can take 10 years off your age, make you look firmer, smoother, and have brighter skin in 24 hours. If these results were possible and long-lasting, we the beauty-obsessed wouldn't be searching any further. The opposite is the case. We are still searching hard, and the ads are selling harder.

"Olay Regenerist Retinol 24. Smoother, brighter, firmer skin in twenty-four hours." If someone were to sell you a pill and said, "Take this! You will run faster, jump higher, and punch stronger in twenty-four hours," I hope you understand the human body enough to have some serious doubts about that claim. Outside of serious illness or injury, our body doesn't change in 24 hours. Our body either changes slowly over time or quickly through a drug that we will pay for dearly later. For the human body, a basic rule to remember is the quicker and stronger the drug's effects, the more (often hidden) its side effects.

"If not using any skincare products (it was initially called *Skin Fasting*) is that good for my skin, why haven't I heard much about it?"

Let's quote what Peter Attia, MD, said on fasting (of food) on his podcast, episode 29.[157] Attia said, "Fasting is the most powerful, simple 'drug' in the toolbox of modern medicine. Why hasn't fasting taken off like the keto diet [or Paleo, vegan, low-carb, Atkins, the Zone, gluten free]? Because no one makes money on this [fasting]." Exactly. No one makes money on a method that advocates no products, purchases, or investments. The media hasn't backed Dr. Utsugi's *Skin Fasting* even though readers in multiple countries have. They aren't likely to back *Skin Sobering* either because there simply isn't any money to be made.

Skin Sobering is not driven by money. *Skin Sobering* is driven by a heartfelt mission of disseminating the truth about skin beauty and skin epidemics.

Many powerhouse writers have delved into the power of noises: promotion and social media. One of them is Cal Newport, author of *Deep Work*, among others. In it, Newport dissects the "any-benefit" mindset in an attempt to convince readers to quit social media like Twitter, Instagram, and Facebook. He urges us to ruthlessly discard any websites that don't inherently contribute to a quality life. Some highlights are:

> I call this way of thinking [justifying a decision] the any-benefit mindset, as it identifies any possible benefit as sufficient justification for using a *network tool*.

> The problem with this approach, of course, is that it ignores all the negatives that come along with the *tools* in question.

> The question once again is not whether *Twitter* offers some benefits, but instead whether it offers enough benefits to offset *its drag on your time and attention* (*two resources* that are especially valuable to a *writer*).

> Or maybe *social media tools* are at the core of your existence. You won't know either way until you sample life without them.[158]

Using skincare products is a great parallel as it perfectly fits the "any-benefit" way of thinking. Let's replace Newport's subject focus from *social media* to *skincare products*. The passages and principle read surprisingly well:

> I call this way of thinking the any-benefit mindset, as it identifies any possible benefit as sufficient justification for using *skincare products*.

> The problem with this approach, of course, is that it ignores all the negatives that come along with the *skincare products* in question.

The question once again is not whether a *moisturizer* offers some benefits, but instead whether it offers enough benefits to offset its *damage to your skin, your time, and your money* (*three resources* that are especially valuable to *everyone*)."

Or maybe *cleansers and masks* are at the core of your existence. You won't know either way until you sample life without them.

Do the benefits outweigh the costs? Before *Skin Sobering*, did you even know there were costs—to your skin!—not just to your wallet?

More powerhouse writers have torn apart the world of products and marketing. In *Sapiens: A Brief History of Humankind*, author Yuval Harari talks about "romantic consumerism," which describes a way of thinking that is incorporated into anything and everything in our lives. Romantic consumerism tells us that "in order to be happy we must consume as many products and services as possible. If we feel that something is missing or not quite right, then we probably need to buy a product or a service. Every television commercial is another little legend about how consuming some product will make life better."[159]

Skin care companies are experts at using romantic consumerism. They have flooded our minds with endless beautiful-looking and -smelling products, so that without them, we don't feel special. Yet, indulging in them makes us the least special because we are just like the other billion people who fell for consumerism and corporate strategy in a desperate search for self-esteem and fulfillment.

PRESENCE, NOT ABSENCE

Our world is also set up to solve simple problems with complicated solutions, thinking of *presence* rather than *absence* as the way to a solution. This way of thinking is for business and the never-ending wheel of the economy. Even though "less is more," people usually feel that more is better. We are too conditioned toward doing something (presence) to solve our problems. We seek intervention too quickly instead of adjusting our habits and lifestyle. When we experience a minor health problem, we feel the need to do something about it, rather than give it time and not interfere. A simple cold can quickly lead to antibiotic use instead of the simpler and effective method of resting and drinking fluids. This "need for stuff" mentality is a big obstacle for *Skin Sobering*, which is the quintessential *absence of products*.

On the other hand, this is the best time to advocate for *Skin Sobering*. People are realizing that natural is better than altered; solar energy is less harmful than fossil fuels; and a simple life is a freer life. More people are fascinated by the time-tested wisdom of the ages—eat what has been around for centuries and use what your great-great-grandmother used. If people are willing to go through the obstacle of complicated diets for better health, would they also be willing to try the simple and no-cost way of *Skin Sobering* for better skin and health?

Ask yourself questions before you consume: Is what I'm buying benefiting me more than it is costing me? Am I buying to fill a need, to feel special, or to curb boredom? Is the person or company selling me a solution or trying to profit? There are no polar answers to any of these questions, but a sliding scale that can help you see where you stand. Now that you know skincare products cause harm and give you temporary visual benefits, exercise some restraint and ask questions before you pay and use them. Break free from the alluring promises of advertising with your new knowledge.

KIM KARDASHIAN OR ROSA PARKS

Skin Sobering will be a hard sell. Even worse, any person or organization who has a financial relationship with this industry will not want this concept to go anywhere. Dr. Utsugi and I may have our credentials questioned or perhaps our reputations smeared. We may have to brace ourselves for one-star reviews by haters and trolls who want everyone to think we are full of crap, so the important information we've tried to share here gets buried. The skincare and cosmetics industry is bigger than the insurance, finance, alcohol, or automotive industries in terms of marketing dollars spent. So, getting the word out about *Skin Sobering* will be a challenge, but we know it is worth it.

In today's digital world, many are convinced that to make a change—to make a difference—one needs all the influencers and promotional help one can get. A 15-year-old daughter of a great friend once lectured me during our dim sum lunch: "Auntie, you need to be famous to have anyone listen to you. You need to have followers to make any difference." Well, Macy is from the Kardashian generation. I, however, am from the Rosa Parks generation.

I believe a few dedicated people with a passion for doing the right thing can make a change.

Here's another story of a dedicated force for good.

Robert Stewart devoted his life to studying and filming sharks. He went undercover to confront the shark fin industry, an industry that collects its product by removing fins from sharks and discarding the rest of the wounded fish back into the ocean, alive. These mutilated sharks eventually die of suffocation because they are unable to swim, and they sink to the bottom of the ocean. Stewart's film, *Sharkwater*, won more than 40 film awards. His follow-up film, *Revolution*, was the highest-grossing Canadian documentary of the year, and it received 19 global awards. Stewart also wrote *Save the Humans*, a biography detailing the importance of sharks in his life and how they make a positive impact in the ocean. In 2016, he launched a Kickstarter campaign to fund *Sharkwater: Extinction*. This film would focus on the 80 million sharks killed per year that are unaccounted for by scientists. Unfortunately, while he was working on the film, Robert Stewart drowned.

In an interview with this fearless warrior fighting this lonely war, Stewart said, "We only need three percent of the population to be totally invested in an issue to change the world." Mothers Against Drunk Driving (MADD), seatbelt and helmet laws, Amber Alerts, Charity Water, Greta Thunberg, taking peanuts out of schools, hockey neck guards, shark-fin bans—whether you support any or all of the above, they all had a small but mighty army behind them, and they succeeded in making a change.

Hey, Macy (who probably doesn't even remember we had this conversation), I don't need to be famous and popular to make a difference. I need 3% of you to care about your skin beauty, health, the environment, and lab animals enough that you care to spread the message of *Skin Sobering*. If our effort is a success, there will be less cosmetic animal testing, less bottles, plastic, and microbeads filling the ocean, and less inflammatory skin disease in children and adults. We can have a cleaner world, a decrease in skin diseases and discomfort, and a celebration of naturally beautiful skin.

14

MY STORY

FROM THE BEAUTY-OBSESSED SCIENTIST

I did not win the skin lottery, nor did I win the birth lottery.

I won the parents lottery.

I was born in 1965 in the remote village of San Yuan (三原) near Xi An (西安), the old capital city in northwest (陕西) China. Shortly after my birth, the infamous Cultural Revolution began. This was a violent sociopolitical movement that lasted 10 years (1966 to 1976). Its goal was to preserve Chinese Communist Party ideals; therefore, all signs of capitalism and traditional historical elements were purged.

My dad, who returned to China from Indonesia to study medicine, was prosecuted for having Western influences. To "reeducate" him, they sent my dad to "study camps" on and off for six years. My mom, who they assumed was his accomplice, had to accompany him on some of these mind-reform journeys. So, I was a wild child without consistent parental care, just like many children of that time. If you had grandparents around, you were golden because you could have home-cooked food. I didn't. So, like everyone else, I ate "black buns" (黑馍馍; hei mo mo)—steam buns made from unprocessed grains—twice a day from our hospital's canteen. We were lucky because we had food, and it was free. And now I know I was indeed lucky, because for the first nine years of my life, I basically just ate plants and only twice a day (accidental healthy habits).

I did get an egg every year on my birthday, which I painted pink and carried in a crochet pouch around my neck for the entire day. I felt so pretty, so I know my beauty obsession started young! The other days, weeks, and months, we kids just roamed around the hospital compound and explored its hidden forest and secret burial grounds. We did some god-awful, innocent things. I was just 6 or 7, and I survived with only some cuts and scrapes, mild bruises, and moderate bullying.

My dad lost his hearing from a forceful slap to his left ear during one of his "reeducate and confess" sessions. I witnessed one of these sessions by climbing up a mud wall barricade, which was spiked with broken glass at the top to prevent snoopers like me. I missed my dad and had decided to go looking for him. I saw what they did to him as I bled from my arms, and from within. My dad saw me, and he didn't just lose his hearing—he lost his trust in people too.

The reported unnatural deaths during the Cultural Revolution range from hundreds of thousands to between 20 and 80 million, depending on what your source is.[160,161] As a frame of reference, Hitler was responsible for 12 million concentration camp deaths, and 30 million other deaths associated with World War II.

My dad, mom, and I survived, and the rest of my childhood journey was a wealth of loving and free-minded parenting. I rarely read as a kid because there was nothing much allowed, and little of what was available was even interesting. I could recite *The Little Red Book*, also known as *Quotations from Chairman Mao Zedong* at a very young age, so my reading job was long done. Interesting things came to me instead through my dad's storytelling and singing. He had a lot of stories and songs, and he sang at a professional level (I later realized this when I heard the professionals).

Neither of my parents were too protective of me. When I was in the village, I was allowed to walk to kindergarten unaccompanied. I didn't really walk, though. I hung on the back of horse buggies for most of the way, usually until the farmer spotted me and beat me off with a long whip. I could play in the rain, snow, and mud with no repercussions. I had a bath only every season in a huge bathhouse with all my friends and our mothers. But every night, my parents would make sure I washed my face, feet, and bum with my own hands. 🎵 洗臉洗腳洗屁股 🎵 (xi lian xi jiao xi pi gu)—essentially all the holes on my body. It was a song my dad made up. I rarely got sick, but when I did, my dad would sit beside me the whole night to monitor my breathing and temperature. My mom was an obstetrician-gynecologist and worked shifts, so my dad wanted her to get her sleep.

When we got to Hong Kong, I was 9, and I was allowed to take the bus to school on my own. That cured my severe motion sickness, a product of me rarely seeing or smelling a motor vehicle until I left my village. At school, I could join any activities—debate club, dance club, choir, Duke of Edinburgh's Award Program, Community Youth Club, drama club, poem recital club, and the volleyball team—and hang out with my friends, as long as I was home for dinner. The dinner rule was firm until I was 19, when I left for Canada. Because of that, I could never have a romantic dinner with my first boyfriend, but he was always at my home for family meals. My boyfriend met all my relatives and had great chef's-quality meals. My dad could cook at a professional level too. I wasn't wildly roaming the village forest anymore, but I was free and busy exploring the metropolitan city of Hong Kong. If you haven't been, it's like New York on steroids. When my dad wasn't working, he would take me everywhere on the bus and show me how the city was run and how people behaved. Again, I did very little reading. I learned most of my living skills from my trusting and free-minded parents.

I could have never imagined that one day I'd write this book, or any book, because I wasn't even a reader (of fiction, I should clarify). Reading stories was deemed by the communists to be "thought-contaminating." My dad's singing and storytelling was brilliant because, unlike written words, sounds left no trace, so no one was able to report us with evidence to the party leaders. Coincidentally, my starting to read novels was also linked to communism, at the age of 36.

The first movie that made me feel the power of writing, and has remained one of my favorites, was *Enemy at the Gates*. If you have not seen it, oh, please do! Jean-Jacques Annaud brilliantly directed this 1973 adaptation of William Craig's nonfiction book of the same name. Most people would say that Vasily Zaytsev, the sniper, was the hero. Who wouldn't fall in love with Vasily, played by the beautiful Jude Law? But the person who truly changed the course of the war and gave the people of this failing nation hope was Commisar Danilov, a lieutenant and a brilliant writer. In the movie, he regularly published encouraging tales in the army's newsletter of Vasily's courageous exploits. The writing painted Vasily as a national hero and bolstered the Russian army's morale. This all led to them eventually winning the battle for the city. The pen was undoubtedly mightier than the sword (or in this case, the rifle).

Ironically, as I digested this story about communist propaganda, something just clicked in my no-longer-communist-brainwashed mind. I realized that reading and writing are far more powerful than brute force. I was a reader, but mostly of academic materials. I read what I needed to earn each of my degrees, and I didn't utilize reading for pleasure or spiritual improvement. I was 36 and knew I had to read more to be better. However, it wasn't until I got to my 50s that I really had the time to read and to improve.

I remember vividly after one long bicycle ride, I said to my husband, Bruce, "I know what I want to do in my fifties." I spent most of my 20s improving my intellect so I would be competitive in the academic world. My 30s revolved around raising my sons with their great dad—training them, educating them, helping them, and bringing the "rice" home. Then came my harder-working 40s, building my businesses and adjusting to a blended family while working so many 18-hour days. All that made me bitchy and intolerant. Now that I'm in my vibrant 50s, I want to be a better version of myself (however cliché that may sound). I want to expand my perspectives, strengthen my relationships, and work on my health.

I told Bruce I needed to read to broaden my viewpoint, to deepen my understanding, and to challenge my tolerance and acceptance, for my sake and for the sake of everyone around me. Bruce hugged me close and, with emotion tightening his throat, he said, "I'm so happy, my love!"

Meeting Dr. Utsugi was a result of reading, which led to my calling in life.

THE BEAUTY-OBSESSED SCIENTIST— FROM SKIN DEEP TO DEEP

SKIN DEEP...

When you have lived half a century (a short time, again according to my 85-year-old mom), you have experienced life. If you know what you want to do by then, you are lucky. I'm thrilled to have developed my true calling so late in life, after many career twists and turns. My calling is beauty and health—to study, practice, write, and disseminate the knowledge and method behind how to be your healthiest and most beautiful self. *I won't have one without the other*—缺一不可 (que yi bu ke).

If something just made my skin healthier, I wouldn't listen. I had given up health for beauty many times throughout my life, which eventually made me not beautiful. No one can turn back the clock, but you don't need to accelerate your aging either. Those who are still young and haven't disrupted their skin to the point of no return still have time to skin sober. You can skin sober no matter what age you are. My mom started it at 82. She has better skin than Jane Fonda.

Even though I wasn't gifted with a win in the skin genetics lottery, my friends now say, "But you *have* nice skin, Erin." Well, bingo! My skin is looking relatively nice now because as people keep damaging their skin, it worsens at a faster speed. My skin's deterioration, on the other hand, has not only slowed down since I began *Skin Sobering*, but some of my aging signs were even reversed. On top of that, what I save from not using skin products has been freeing. *Skin Sobering* freed me up to think of and do other things that are good for me and people who matter to me. I read books and write. I cook more, exercise more, and see friends more. I've saved so much money not just on the regular seasonal "restock fees" for all my go-to products, but on the here-and-there impulse purchases of "hope" when I run by the store for romaine lettuce, durian, or fresh corn—which is frequently. All of my new habits helped me to decelerate my aging. My skin at 57 has maintained its good functioning and is looking quite fine compared to others my age or younger.

We believe everyone can benefit from *Skin Sobering*, but the biggest impact will likely be for people between 30 and 60 years old. As we've already discussed, in our teens and 20s, we often feel invincible. We want to explore and rebel. Between our 30s and 60s, we have finally tried enough, failed enough, and are humble enough. When we want to pamper ourselves, we want to be smart about it. By this time, we have also matured, and we care about more than just ourselves. We think of the environment, ethics, our actions, and who we are responsible for besides ourselves.

In our 30s, many of us have babies and young children who can't take care of themselves. Their largest organ's health and overall well-being are in our hands. Our knowledge affects us and our offspring. Starting in our 50s, we face another overwhelming responsibility: caring for our parents. Many of them are embarking upon their end-of-life journey and are suffering as their ability to care for themselves deteriorates. So, we are responsible for their health and care.

Our knowledge and actions don't just affect us alone anymore.

I learned this the hard way.

...TO DEEP

Beauty and health are my two favorite subjects. I will dive into them whether I'm writing a book or not. Since I paid so much attention to beauty, I was also brainwashed quite deeply by the beauty industry. It's one thing to realize I was hurting my own skin with products, it's another to know that my dad's skin was tormented by me.

When my dad became terminally ill in 2018, my mom and I became his arms and legs. We cared for him in every way, feeding him, cleaning him, and helping him with his most primitive bodily functions. My mom did the lion's share of the work, followed by my eldest son, Yang Yang, and my husband. Carrying a 200-pound weak body wasn't something my mom and I could do. Thank God for my on-demand, loving sons and husband.

When my dad's condition worsened, he lost everything that defined him. He could no longer sing, tell stories, or even turn himself in bed. In the depths of his despair, he begged us to have him euthanized, and he asked that we keep him at home. We didn't have the power or the heart to do the former, but we honored the latter till his last breath. He was a proud man who wanted to be in control, so he controlled his eating and voiding and did neither much in his last months. But my mom and I still controlled his cleaning, out of love.

Out of love, we washed my dad daily with chemicals to keep him *smelling* clean, and we lathered his back with moisturizers because I thought they would help ease his dry skin. The two places we couldn't do our cleaning deeds were his face and chest—he would swat my hands away to protect his front, but he couldn't protect his back.

My Baba cried over his itchy back until his last day. He had no problem with his face and chest. If only I knew what I know now...I am so sorry, Ba.

I think if someone chooses to do anything to their own body, at least one can say, "You had a choice, and maybe you were misinformed, but it was your own choice based on what you knew." The same concept doesn't apply to those of us taking care of the young or the old, both of whom are vulnerable and have no choice. So, our knowledge becomes even more crucial because of our responsibilities for our loved ones—not just for ourselves.

I need to give people the truth, even in the face of the huge conglomerates who would rather keep it hidden and keep me quiet.

Skin Sobering wasn't really started as a quest for personal beauty. It was started as a personal mission to convince one person at a time to walk away from the train wreck that is skincare products. End the self-inflicted beauty issues, end the skin problem epidemic, and end another vulnerable person's pointless suffering!

TIME TO COME CLEAN

Here are the things I've done to my body in the name of vanity, most of which have been in vain. I've used a lot of skincare products, starting with small amounts in my mid-20s. When money wasn't so tight with raising kids, I went all out with a lot more types and higher price points. I told myself that I worked hard and deserved to treat my skin. I also had injections, chemical and light treatments—IPL, Botox, fillers, hyaluronidase to dissolve fillers, Halo, micro laser peels, Thermage, BBL (BroadBand Light), and Clear & Brilliant—in the 20-plus years that I was obsessed with beauty.

I had braces as an adult to correct a class 3 malocclusion (underbite); composite bonding on my incisor to restore a chipped tooth from a childhood playground swing accident and tetracycline-stained teeth (a common antibiotic that caused graying teeth in children who grew up in China in the '60s and '70s). I also had breast implants to restore my completely flattened breasts after breastfeeding my three sons, each for six months to one year. Breastfeeding doesn't do that to every woman. My mom still has full breasts at age 85. My grandma, on the other hand, like me also had "envelope breasts"—my mom called them that—after breastfeeding. The "syndrome" skipped a generation with my mom and was passed down to me. So, I think fat and volume loss is more due to genetics than the act of breastfeeding. I don't ever want to discourage breastfeeding. It was a convenient, healthy, and beautiful experience for me.

Skincare products didn't resolve any of the problems for which they were marketed. When the products were on, my skin was briefly plumper and less dry. As soon as the products were off, all my skin problems reappeared. Some of them had gotten worse. After I stopped using skincare products (including cleansers), all my skin problems improved, and many went away completely. The improvements were gradual. Some were noticeable after a couple of weeks, and some took a month or two. And after a year, most of the things that were supposed to be fixed by products had repaired themselves with *Skin Sobering*.

There are unexpected bonuses as well. For example, my wounds and blemishes heal faster with no scarring, and the whites of my eyes are whiter because no chemicals are sneaking in there causing irritation and inflammation, which leads to pigmentation problems. I think a few of the more invasive facial treatments did do my skin some good in some respects, but they also made my skin thin, weak, and sensitive. Thank goodness I didn't do these treatments as frequently as I was urged to by the medi-spa physician and nurses. I would definitely be a *thin-skinned* and *oversensitive* person.

15

YOUR WAY

SKINCARE PRODUCTS ARE LIKE DRUGS, TREATS, AND MAKEUP—DON'T USE THEM EVERY DAY

KNOW YOUR TRUE SKIN

TAKE IT UP A NOTCH
PASS—Protect. Adjust. Skin Sober.

SOBER SKIN ASSESSMENT

HOW TO KEEP SKIN SOBERING GOING AND GOING FAR

FROM THE BEAUTY-OBSESSED SCIENTIST

"Are we becoming too paranoid of bad substances? Now we can't even use cleansers and creams? In the good old days, people drank cola, ate chips, and enjoyed sugar! Now these are all apparently poisonous to our health. Can't we live a little anymore?"

To that argument, Michael Pollan said, we must remember that back in the "good old days," life was not so abundant. Families only had processed "food-like" products as *treats*, like during holidays, festivals, and birthdays. Otherwise, they ate real food; they ate the things they grew and harvested. Now? Supply is so ample that heavily processed products are no longer rare treats. They are eaten daily and multiple times a day. Soda has replaced water, and people drink it whenever they want. Frequency is the problem.[162]

Skincare and cosmetic products are the same. In the old days, they were used sparingly, like one thin layer for a special occasion. There also wasn't an endless sea of options to choose from. Even though women have been putting substances on their skin for thousands of years,[163] they could only very occasionally enhance their skin. Further, only those who were affluent could afford to do it, similar to the sugar situation. In general, most women's skin was bare, undisturbed, and *unprotected*—two out of three ain't bad. Now, we use between 2 to 16 types of different products 24/7. When skincare products are used occasionally, the bad effects can't accumulate and the temporary benefit can be enjoyed, just like sugar. The way we use them now, along with spas and home treatments, we ensure the negative effects won't go away.

Anything we do infrequently is not going to do much harm or good to us. If you smoke once a year or even once a month, no biggie—your lungs will recover. If you binge exercise or eat tons of vegetables once a month, no luck—you are not going to be healthier. Health cannot be achieved in a day or two; illness also requires long periods of destruction. Skin damage is cumulative. There's no one skincare product or bad behavior that will age your skin overnight. Skin "care" is cumulative too. There's not one trick or product that will transform your skin in 24 hours. It is consistency and persistence that lead to change. Time is a magical thing.

KNOW YOUR TRUE SKIN

Here's one more reason to start *Skin Sobering*. If you learn nothing else, *Skin Sobering* is the only way to know the true condition of this important organ. Many skin issues are caused by skin care and lifestyle habits. If you want to find out the causes of your skin problems, don't mask them with skincare or makeup products. Leave your skin alone and give it enough time to recuperate from product disruptions first. Your skin will show you how well or bad off it really is, and in time it will learn how to behave properly again.

When you first start, please don't obsess over your skin for the first 7 to 14 days. I know how hard it is not to study its every transition and cry about every undesirable change. The more you have depended on products, the worse the changes are going to be for the first couple of weeks. That is normal, just like quitting smoking. You are training your body.

After 14 days, assess your skin's condition. Your skin has been so confused due to the constant product and environmental beatings it has endured, and skin types are so often misclassified. Even bra fitting—a much simpler task—is done wrong by 80% of women, so imagine the complexity of skin. Your skin has its own innate characteristics, but it has been altered by products for too long. So, oily skin may feel like dry skin because you frequently strip your oil off with cleansers; normal skin may feel like sensitive skin because it's reacting to chemicals you apply; dry skin may actually just be normal if it isn't smeared with creams that inhibit its own oil production; acne-prone skin is just young skin that is going through a hormonal phase and can heal quickly on its own; itchy skin may be chemically assaulted skin that is fighting back.

Even the simple benefit of really knowing your skin and its condition is a nice perk of *Skin Sobering*. Knowing your true skin will help you buy the right skincare products, right? And you may just find out how much better your skin is after your skin sobers up for 30 days.

TAKE IT UP A NOTCH

Skin Sobering is for whom? It's for mature people who have tried everything, for teens who are troubled by more than their acne, for picky women who know all their flaws, for parents who care for their young children, and for sons and daughters who need to know how to protect their frail parents. *Skin Sobering* is also for men who have dry or oily skin, itchy scalps, dandruff, or nongenetic hair thinning. We all have been brainwashed to believe that skin care means cleansing with products, moisturizing with products, improving with products, and protecting with products. Those are all profit-driven messages. Our skin can do its own work way better than any products, if we just let it.

Let nature do what it does best. Your NMF is your moisturizer. Don't strip it away. Your bricks and mortar are your protective barrier. Don't break them down. Your symbiotic bacteria are your best friends. Don't kill them off. Your sweat and oil feed those symbiotic friends. Don't starve them. Your natural cell exfoliation is your skin's best method of renewal. Don't mess it up.

That's a solid list of Don'ts, so now some Dos to pass down!

PASS—PROTECT. ADJUST. SKIN SOBER.

P for Protect

How our skin looks to the world has largely been decided by our genetics and our culture. We can't control these two things. Putting genetics and cultural perception aside, to have *your* best, most beautiful skin, your immediate responsibility is to (P) protect it. Protect your face from the sun and harsh elements. The best and most extreme approach is avoidance. Many of my Asian friends whose priority is to have fair skin have as little exposure to the sun as possible. They live an indoor life with their windows covered with blinds. They do not go out during daytime, and they use sunscreens day and night. That is excessive, especially the last part.

I want physical fitness, and I love exercising *and* beautiful skin, so I resort to the second-best protection: physical shields. I walk in the shade and use hats, umbrellas, and sports masks during long physical activities. I am known as the "cover girl" or "bandit" in my cycling group, depending on if they think my look is hot or hideous. The face mask not only protects me against UV rays, but it also shields me from wind, dust, bugs, and dirt. With skiing, wearing a balaclava is as necessary as wearing goggles, so my quirkiness is common on the slopes. So find yourself a shielding gadget that keeps the sun away from your face, and exercise away on sunny, shady, and stormy days.

Sunscreen products do some negative things to the skin, but compared to harmful UV rays, they are the lesser of two evils. Use them if you really can't shield your face. A little indirect sunlight is better for you than a lot of sunscreen. Always wash off your sunscreen as soon as you are done with your outdoor activity.

A for Adjust

To (A) adjust your lifestyle is not easy, and it is an ever-evolving effort. Not smoking, drinking less, sleeping well, exercising regularly, and eating better all require willpower and discipline. You must have the willpower to start, to continue, and to persist until you see results.

Since I started *Skin Sobering*, I have gained three extra hours a day. How? These are hours that I am no longer spending putting on and taking off products. I have hundreds of dollars more a month to put into savings or to spend on other things, and I have twice the brain space to focus on better things. At first, I added a 7-minute, full-body workout. Now that has turned into 50 minutes with weights and yoga on alternate days. In addition to my seasonal cycling and skiing, I did some fads like hula-hooping, rope jumping, and belly dancing. Recently, I added playing pickleball, six days a week. So addictive. Since I had the time to try more things, I'm now loving making my own fermented foods (kombucha, kimchi, sauerkraut, Chinese cabbage, and sticky rice), and cooking all my food. I connect with family and friends more, and I had the time to write this book!

Lifestyle changes require constant adjusting and readjusting, not deprivation or *3-minute passion* 三分鐘熱度 (san fen zhong re du)—literally a 3-minute, heated urge that doesn't last. We have a saying in Chinese (of course we do)—*the new toilet even gets more poop* 新屎坑三日香 (xin shi keng san ri xiang), meaning, anything that's new will get more attention and use. When you are gung-ho to drop a bad habit, you likely will be psyched and want nothing of it, for a while. Deprivation, to me, doesn't work. It is like holding my breath underwater: sooner or later, I won't be able to take it. Lifestyle changes are not easy, and they need to be lifelong to have real benefits. Replacement rather than deprivation worked for me. I replaced red bean taro bubble tea with kombucha, meat with unlimited tasty veggies, scrolling Instagram posts with reading a good book, and I swapped out chips for nuts. All these took time and willpower to do, which I gained because *Skin Sobering* simplified my life.

To give your skin what it needs in terms of *lifestyle* adjustment is not easy to achieve. It took me and my husband six years to get to a food-fasting level where our bodies are benefiting from autophagy, insulin regulation, and caloric control. We learned the wrong things, we failed, and we started again, a little bit at a time. We persisted, and now we eat real food, we don't eat too frequently, and we enjoy it all—especially plants—about 80% of the time. Being a B+ to A- student is good enough.

Being perfect is painful.

I understand that making these healthy lifestyle changes may strike some people as drastic and radical. Maybe so, but a life of needles, injections, surgeries, micro lasers, chemical peels, Photoshop, Instagram filters, endless product trial and error, refills and acquisition, and multi-hour, twice-daily skincare routines sound much more drastic and radical to me.

SS for Skin Sober

I don't need to reiterate the way of *Skin Sobering* anymore, but I want to share with you the many mistakes I made in the process of *Skin Sobering*—and I have read Dr. Utsugi's original book plus dozens of other skin books. Imagine a less experienced person trying to do this right.

When I first started practicing *Skin Sobering*, I would scratch my chin and above my lips every time I showered to make sure the dead skin was gone. I knew chemicals were bad, but I thought I could mechanically exfoliate with my fingertips—I forgot entirely that scrubbing and rubbing are bad, let alone scratching. The more I scratched, the flakier my skin got. That area became even drier and more vulnerable, but my cheeks and forehead were smooth and glowy, from just gently washing them with water. Once I stopped scratching, the problem stopped.

Again, your face only needs water, no soap. Your hands, groin, and armpits can take pure soap daily because the hands touch toilets, and groins and armpits have big, oily glands.

I also was worried that my face and body were not clean enough. I have a deep-seated obsession with cleanliness, too, so I increased my washing time and the temperature. I figured longer washes and hotter temperatures ought to kill more bad germs. Neither one helped my skin condition. I went to bed with itchy skin until I learned to lower the water temperature and shortened my shower time. Recently, I started practicing what I affectionately call "Wim-py Hof." Wim Hof, also known as "The Iceman," is a motivational speaker and athlete known for his ability to withstand freezing temperatures. I call it "Wim-py" when I do it, because I'm not diving into ice baths, but I do take quite cold showers. My itching completely went away, and my skin is even more hydrated. That's the power of water and temperature in both the negative and positive directions.

I also made mistakes with my makeup application. I use a loose mineral powder foundation to even my skin tone when I go out. This light layer is illuminating, especially on the smooth skin I regained after *Skin Sobering*. The powder washes off with just water, so I love it. However, at first, after I brushed the powder on, I often saw dry skin flakes mixed in with the powder as if my skin was peeling. This was perplexing because I didn't feel dry at all. It took me a year (actually 12 makeup applications) to realize that the way I used the brush itself was incorrect. I used a heavy rotary motion to buff the powder, believing the pressure and friction would make the powder blend better with my skin. I was literally "mopping" my face with the brush. The brush was basically prematurely exfoliating the top layer of my stratum corneum, hence the flakes. When I stopped buffing and mopping and just used feathery strokes to apply the powder, my skin was smooth and luminous—no more flakes!

SOBER SKIN ASSESSMENT

Skin Sobering may be simple, but because we have so many preconceived, deep-seated ideas and misinformation about our skin, we run into more and different issues. In order to execute *Skin Sobering* accurately so you feel confident and your skin recovers the fastest, we developed a tool called the *Sober Skin Assessment (SSA)* to give you some metrics about your skin before and after *Skin Sobering*, and your future skin.

A chemical-free life with zero outside damage and zero poor lifestyle habits produces the most desirable skin life. So, a score of zero and a face that is flawless is the best, but impossible to achieve for us mere mortals. However, the opposite of this—full-blown damage represented by a score of 100 and a face full of stains—is possible to avoid (Figure H). The *SSA* will yield two metrics—a *Skin Score*, and a *Face Chart*—which can reveal your skin condition, provide a record for your baseline, and help monitor your skin's progress before and after *Skin Sobering*. The lower the *Skin Score* and clearer the *Face Chart*, the better

Figure H

A sample illustration of a Skin Score of 0, and a Face Chart of "Flawless" (don't aim for perfection); versus one of a Skin Score of 100 and a Face Chart of "Disaster." (Hope you don't destroy your skin like that!)

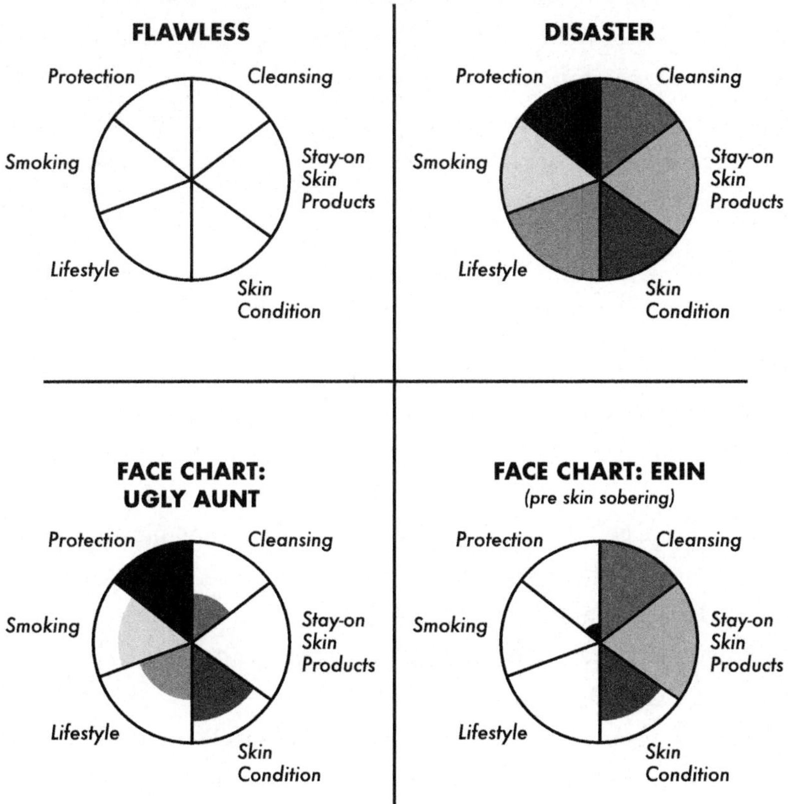

FLAWLESS

DISASTER

FACE CHART: UGLY AUNT

Skin Score = 68.5

Not much chemical damage, severe UV damage, moderate lifestyle issues.

We predict her skin will age faster than people her age.

FACE CHART: ERIN
(pre skin sobering)

Skin Score = 50.5

Maximum chemical damage from cleansing and leave-on products, minimal UV damage and lifestyle issues.

We predict her skin will age at a similar rate as people her age.

YOUR WAY • 275

your skin. The *SSA* can also give you insight into your future skin, predicting how healthy and beautiful your skin will be based on what you do now. Please visit *www.skinsobering.ca/soberskinassessment* to get your free assessment and report.

The *Skin Sobering* book will give you sufficient knowledge and skills to be a lifelong skin soberer. Many people can quit a bad habit or adopt a healthy way of living on their own after they understand and make the decision to just do it. It is the same for *Skin Sobering*. But if you want more assistance than this book, to receive a clinical assessment, monitoring, and feedback on your skin, please visit our free self-help program at *www.skinsobering.ca*.

HOW TO KEEP SKIN SOBERING GOING AND GOING FAR

If you agree with us and understand all the good that quitting skin products can do for your health and beauty, spread the word! Massive corporations will undoubtedly want to shut us up; small boutiques will wish this concept never crossed the Pacific Ocean; and big-shot beauty professionals, influencers, and even megastars may try to silence our healthy, sober skin message. We need your help to get the message out, as real-world experience and word of mouth will likely be our only means to share our message.

Nobel Prize recipient Francis Crick once said, "Politeness is the poison of all good collaboration in science...A good scientist values criticism almost higher than friendship: no, in science criticism is the height and measure of friendship." This is true, but when you criticize something, you must speak from a position of knowledge and facts, not headlines and hype. You must also equip yourself with understanding and kindness (different from politeness), not emotional outbursts or takedowns. Above all, you must always endeavor to back up your opinions with good science. That's when learning, exchanging, enrichment, and improvement happens.

The skin care debate is heating up, and we think *Skin Sobering* should be part of the conversation. We welcome discussion, critique, and debate, and we're looking forward to hearing what real people have to say after they've given this simple solution a try. Message us!

Our effort is grassroots, one book at a time, one reader at a time, and one believer at a time.

conclusion

For the better part of a century, we've been led to believe that our face or skin cannot be beautiful and healthy without skincare products. Billions of dollars every year are spent to convince us of that fallacy. We've been told that all our germs and our own secretions are bad, so we use cleansers that invariably strip away our skin's natural protections, leaving it vulnerable. To counteract this, we then attempt to rehydrate it and add "nutrients" back by applying even more chemicals. Yet our skin is an excretory organ, an impermeable protective barrier designed to get rid of waste and to *keep things out*. Forcing our skin to absorb moisture and nutrients is just a mockery of nature.

Skin Sobering uses science, evidence, and a woman's desire to be beautiful to evoke change.

So, one more time for the people in the back: **skincare products are not necessary for beauty and health. They are damaging to your skin. Skincare products create the very problems they claim to solve while offering temporary, visual, or tactile enhancements, just like makeup does.** If this knowledge is disseminated and adopted, *Skin Sobering* will "save your skin" just like quitting smoking can save your life.

Dr. Utsugi and I did not write *Skin Sobering* for the sole purpose of discussing beauty. "Beauty" is merely the flag we wave to grab your attention because there is so much more to it. Beneath the "skin-deep" issue of beauty is a hidden war, an ever-increasing epidemic of skin health and diseases. Eczema, dermatitis, allergies, irritation, and other skin problems that are too medically serious for beauty books to address are not attracting the attention of beauty-conscious readers. On the other hand, dryness, oiliness, acne, fine lines, wrinkles, puffiness, dull skin, and sensitivity—conditions that are only skin-deep—are being dismissed by traditional scientists as shallow. But both the "serious" and the "shallow" are connected to chemicals on the skin: skincare products.

In 2021, billionaire Bernard Arnault beat Amazon's Jeff Bezos and took the throne of the richest person in the world for a while. And what does Mr. Arnault own? LVMH, which owns globally prestigious brands like Louis Vuitton, Moët, and Hennessy, as well as luxury skincare brands like Acqua di Parma, Benefit Cosmetics, Cha Ling, Fresh, Givenchy, Guerlain, Kendo Brands of BITE Beauty, Fenty Beauty by Rihanna, Marc Jacobs Beauty, KVD Vegan Beauty, Ole Henriksen, most high-end perfumes, and of course, Sephora.

The skincare and beauty industry is led by one of the world's richest and most powerful men. How can we be heard over the sheer marketing noise created by billions and billions of dollars? Dr. Utsugi and I are ready to try because we have to. We have science on our side, and now you do too. Join us in shouting about the power of *Skin Sobering* until the skin "care" industry has no choice but to genuinely start caring about the health of our skin.

TIME WILL TELL

The cosmetic industry as we know it is still young.[164] It has only been around in its modern form for about 80 years. The skincare and makeup craze flooding the general public has existed for an even shorter period of time. In comparison, skin has existed naturally for millions of years. What is the best way to know if you have done something right or wrong? Time. Time will tell if you have done the right things for your skin, your body, your relationships, your mind, and the environment. I would like to share one last pearl of Chinese wisdom: *distance shows a horse's strength, time reveals a person's character* 路遙知馬力, 日久見人心 (lu yao zhi ma li, ri jiu jian ren xin). Your skin is made worse by 99% of the products you use. Instead of trying to mask and address the symptoms, try removing the source of the problems—and give it time.

Now you know what your skin needs and wants to be beautiful and stay beautiful. We hope *Skin Sobering* empowers you to fight for your best self and slow your aging down gracefully. Take matters into your own hands, trust the science, and resist the marketing. *Skin Sobering* is *not* like any other self-improvement resolution where you have to invest in something (time to exercise, money to buy healthy foods, energy to declutter and KonMari your junk, skills to cook, etc.). *Skin Sobering* is one of the very few health practices that offers genuine simplicity: allow water and your body a chance to work their miracles.

The end

...OF ALL THE SECRETS!

There is a long list of reasons—physiological, anatomical, chemical, biological, psychological, emotional, legal, and cultural—why skincare products are one of the biggest causes of our skin's beauty and health problems. We've claimed that *Skin Sobering* is your best skin care and beautifying method. *Skin Sobering* is backed by personal experience, evidence, and of course, science, though it can be a lot of information to digest. Below is a list of key points for easy reference, in case you or a loved one ever need it:

1. Skin beauty is primarily determined by genetics, then dictated by cultural perception. See how much someone's skin has *improved*, not just how it *is* (maybe they're born with it) to help you weigh the merits of their recommendation.

2. The skin is an *excretory* and *protective* organ. Its main functions are to excrete waste and create a barrier between you and the world.
    a. Any organ that's designed to excrete (poop) does not want to absorb (eat). We dare not block the anus or

urethra openings, so why do we obstruct with goo and goop the millions of tiny excretory openings on our skin—our pores?

b. Any organ that is created to protect you doesn't want things to get through it. If anything has to be absorbed *through* the skin, that thing has broken down your skin's barrier. Your skin is then injured and leaky. Moisture escapes and dryness ensues.

3. Skincare companies created an entire class of entertainment in the 1940s—soap operas—to sell cleansers and detergents to housewives.

4. P&G was the world's largest single advertiser, spending *$11.5 billion a year* in marketing to convince people that they need products. Its competitors did the same.

5. Our desire to be hygienic has morphed into an obsession with cultural acceptance and a widespread skin problem epidemic.

6. Prior to the 1940s, eczema affected only 5% of children. Its prevalence increased five times by 2007. Other allergic symptoms like asthma, hay fever, and food allergies—the atopic march—have also soared. These all stem from skin irritation, which is strongly linked to using skincare products, natural or synthetic.

7. Cleansers are part of skincare products. Whether they claim to be organic, natural, or synthetic—all are processed products.

8. What we see as "our skin" is the stratum corneum and its corneocytes (the bricks). Together with the intercellular lipid substance (the mortar), they form the skin's protective "bricks and mortar." This "mortar" also has a dual "lipid-water-lipid-water" configuration, making it a great moisture barrier.

9. The stratum corneum must be allowed to naturally exfoliate in order to signal cell renewal. When the skin is clear and fresh, stratum corneum surface cells naturally flake off every three to four days—the best form of exfoliation to achieve smoothness. Products soak the skin and inhibit natural exfoliation. Manual or chemical exfoliation hurt the skin and *cannot* trigger the signaling of new cell production. Your skin ends up thin and coarse *because of* products.

10. The skin's own natural moisturizing factor (NMF) has powerful barrier and moisturizing functions. Skincare companies spend millions in R&D to try to mimic the NMF's functions only to fall severely short. Cleansers strip the NMF away, and moisturizers have less than 1% of NMF's power—*and* they disrupt your skin at the same time.

11. Symbiotic microorganisms protect the skin like an army. They also form the acid mantle and teach the immune system to discriminate between good and harmful microbes. Skin products contain preservatives and more, which can eliminate *all* microbes, killing your skin army.

12. Surfactants, a type of emulsifier, are present in all liquid and viscous forms of products. Surfactants are amphiphilic (water and lipids loving), and are used to make the products smooth

and creamy. This ability will dissolve the "bricks and mortar" and NMF, rendering your skin leaky and dry.

    a. Surfactants and more will get into your pores. The skin rejects these foreign substances by getting inflamed and trying to heal. If product use is not stopped, the inflame-heal-inflame cycle repeats, resulting in a chronic condition. This reoccurring inflammation stimulates melanin precipitation and causes hyperpigmented spots.

13. Oils (essential or synthetic) don't contain surfactants, but they are no better. They are lipophilic, so they can dissolve the "mortar" and damage NMF, leaving your skin dehydrated—from having oil on it!

    a. The long-term use of oils causes an "oil-sunning phenomenon," which is characterized by hyperpigmentation, dullness, and thinning skin, just like the effects of getting too much sun.

14. Cleansing is an integral part of any skincare routine, but cleaning *with products* is harmful to the skin because of the high quantity of surfactants. Surfactants can remove stubborn makeup, but also the acid mantle, microbiome, and NMF—in other words, your entire moisture barrier. Cleansing with products is the first culprit of dry and dehydrated skin.

15. In order for the skin to look different, skincare products have to alter the skin's structure. That is the very definition of a drug according to FDA regulations. Yet skincare products are so loosely regulated that skincare companies can claim anything as long as their wording is vague.

16. The FDA's role is to approve safety, not efficacy. So, the FDA says nothing about whether a product actually does what it claims. The onus is on the beauty company, who has a huge economic incentive and conflict of interest!

17. A common initial reaction to *Skin Sobering* is, unfortunately, dryness. This is the evidence of how your skin has been altered and what it is addicted to. Think of this exactly like the withdrawal effect from quitting a drug—you may feel worse before you feel better, but it's worth it.

18. Inflammation has a profound effect on skin health and aging. "Inflamm-aging" causes skin sensitivity and diseases. Inflammation accelerates aging, and irritation leads to inflammation. What causes irritation? Skincare products!

19. Skincare products are not as bad as drugs, but they are as bad as sugar. Sugar use has increased twentyfold over the last three centuries, as has obesity, diabetes, heart disease, and liver disease. Skincare product use has soared since the advent of the infamous soap opera genre, as has eczema, sensitivity, inflammation, and skin beauty issues.

20. Sixty-nine percent of US women report having sensitive skin. Sensitive skin is not trivial; it is reactive, itchy, and inflamed. It is a medical problem waiting to explode.

21. Skin problems are not minor. Almost 80 million Americans see their doctors about their skin. This outnumbers anxiety, depression, back pain, and diabetes as the *number one* reason Americans see their doctors.

THE END

22. After you have successfully sobered up your skin, you can use skincare products for occasional enhancements, like makeup. Skincare products have essentially the same chemical composition as makeup, just without the color. They both make your skin look good temporarily, but over time, they slowly and surely erode your skin.

we want to hear from you!

Skin Sobering is one book that will leave you with more time, energy, and money than before. Tell us how you are doing! We look forward to celebrating your beautiful results with you! Find us on social media: *@skinsobering*, *#skinsobering*, and *info@skinsobering.com*.

acknowledgments

I need to first thank my oldest friend, Jackie Tsang (and the entourage of GFGHGL—Good Friends Good Health Good Life). Jackie was the one who brought Dr. Utsugi's book to me at our annual dinner in Hong Kong and urged me to try *Skin Sobering*. I rated Jackie as the prettiest one among all my old friends, to which my wonderful editor Jennifer Glover said, "Maybe you should just say *one of the pretty ones*." I replied, "We Chinese have been ranked since birth, so we are thick-skinned and used to the judgment." Besides, people have said that Jackie and I looked alike since we were 11-year-olds, so, there! Jackie is the prettiest one.

Naturally, next is my editor, Jenn. I could not have had a more encouraging and capable editor, one who was also not afraid to hurt my feelings rather than let me publish something bad. She did it so skillfully that my feelings were never hurt, and instead I was invigorated. I admire your tact and talent, Jenn. Another unofficial editor is my stepdaughter, Maggie. Maggie has many talents, and the least known one to her is her editing skills. She balanced law school, a business, and editing my book so effortlessly. Maggie was also the first beautiful young woman who adopted *Skin Sobering* fully and became even more beautiful.

My five sons must also be mentioned because they are my darling boys. My youngest, Alex (昊 Hao Hao—*Horizon*), did almost as much editing, using a (pre)corporate lawyer's perspective, but didn't want any money for it. How unlike a corporate lawyer! Hopefully law school won't change that (at least not for your mama). My musically brilliant oldest and second boys, Aaron (陽 Yang Yang—*Sunshine*) and Andrew (天 Tian Tian—*Ski*) made my audiobook happen, and Tian Tian (the professional singer songwriter) oversaw the entire recording process. How lucky that I can record in the comfort of my pajamas and bare skin, thanks to my gifted sons. My stepson, Wesley, was the person who pioneered *Skin Sobering* in our family without even knowing how beneficial it is. Wesley has the most beautiful hair and skin, a credit to the initial motivation of "no money, no fuss." Jerrel, our oldest, helped give us the most mind-calming gift of making our outdoor sauna work. How many nights when I was stuck and the sauna helped get my creative juices going.

My mama, who's everywhere in this book, who with my Baba gave me everything to become who I am. You are also my oldest skin soberer, with skin better than Jane Fonda and Audrey Hepburn.

I am so fortunate to have many friends to walk along with me on the unfamiliar path of writing and publishing this first book. Nicole H, Kyoko Y, Janice M, Jim C, Lydia C, Shelley L, ex-mom Sue, Jen F, Ademola A, Ho Sir, Yung K, Lan C, Ming W, Sara L, Katelyn H, Wendy C, Jamie C, Mark H, Monica S, Lisa R, Gillian L, Vicki K, Cleo N, and oh, a few more that I might have missed, so sorry. You helped me with my content, my table of contents, my titles, my covers, my outfits, my doubts, and my celebrations. Having friends to experience things together makes everything better. How can I forget my photographer and friend, Jay Parson? You are the best, and you always make me look more beautiful than I feel.

My two doctors, Channy Muhn and Mel Cescon, thank you for assuring me that my science is solid and my mission is meaningful.

And my wonderful publisher, Scribe Media, and your people (in the order that I met you, all superb at your jobs)—Miles Rote, Hal Clifford, Mayra Gonzalez, Katie Villalobos, Erik van Mechelen, Chip Blake, Ron Anahaw, Liz Driesbach, Braxton Benes, Elizabeth Oliver, and Candace Sinclair. And a few more who contributed to my book after I had to lock the manuscript and wasn't allowed to add anything else. You are top-notch in your profession in efficiency, quality, competence, influence, and certainly outcome and human relations. I could not have had a more satisfying and engaging experience. The labor pain is not even over yet with this first baby, and I'm already wanting a second one with you.

And my debt and gratitude to Ryuichi is beyond words. You gave me beautiful and healthy skin to show off. You gave me time and money to do more. You gave me simplicity and clarity to grow further. And you gave me this book. There is more we can do in beauty and health!

Finally, my Bruce, who is also everywhere in my book, and everything to me—brilliant, wise, mature, patient, grumpy, quiet, interesting, fun, boring, handsome, sexy, strong, stubborn, capable, dependable, forgetful, and romantic (this one is getting random and inconsistent)—and the love of my life! My Ba is my fuel to write this book, and you are my reason to live this life!

appendix
FOR CHINESE SAYINGS

Chinese Characters (Pronunciation: Putonghua/Mandarin Pinyin; Cantonese transcription)—*italicized Chinese meaning*. English meaning.

INTRODUCTION

自食其果 (zi shi qi guo; ji sik kei gwo)—*eat their own bad fruit*. They are getting a taste of their own medicine.

自作自受 (zi zuo zi shou; ji jok ji sau)—*self-inflicted, so it serves you right*. They brought the issues on themselves.

CHAPTER 1: REALIZATION

雷聲大雨點小 (lei sheng da yu dian xiao; lieu seng daai yu dim siu)—*big thunder no rain*. Overpromise, underdeliver.

CHAPTER 2: EVIDENCE

乾爽 / 清爽 (gan shuang /qing shuang; gon song/ching song)—*dry fresh*. Clear, fresh, sober skin.

CHAPTER 3: DISBELIEF

蒙在鼓里 (meng zai gu li; mung joi gu lieu)—*wrapped inside the darkness of a big drum.* Kept us in the dark.

苦口良藥 (ku kou liang yao; fu hau leung yeuk)—*good herbal medicine tastes bitter.* Honest advice hurts your feelings.

CHAPTER 4: (BIO)CHEMISTRY

青黃不接 (qing huang bu jie; ching wong bat jip)—*the growing green crop can't catch up to the depleting yellow reserves.* A period of temporary off-balance, off-kilter.

傷口撒鹽 (shang kou sa yan; seung hau saat yim)—*sprinkle salt on the wound.* Add insult to injury.

冰凍三尺非一日之寒 (bing dong san chi fei yi ri zhi han; bing dung saam chek fei yat yat ji hon)—*three feet of ice did not come from one day's cold.* The harm is not from a few days of doing the wrong thing. It's from daily and long-term harm.

CHAPTER 7: PROBLEMS

拔苗助長 (ba miao zhu zhang; bat miu jo jeung)—*pulling the seedlings to help them grow faster.* Your help is essentially killing them faster.

一白遮三醜 (yi bai zhe san chou; yat baak je saam chau)—*one white covers three uglies.* Fair skin is so beautiful that it's enough to hide three ugly facial features.

楚楚可憐 (chu chu ke lian; cho cho ho lin)—*adorable and pitiful!* So delicate and vulnerable, a symbol of beauty.

CHAPTER 8: GUIDE

一步登天 (yi bu deng tian; yat bou dang tin)—*reach the sky in one step.* Build Rome in one day.

296 · SKIN SOBERING

CHAPTER 10: LIFESTYLE

白切雞 (bai zhan ji; baak chit gai)—*bland-steamed chicken.* Free-range, yellow-skin, firm-muscle chicken, steamed or dipped in boiled water, one of the old-time favorites in Chinese cuisine.

熱氣 (re qi; yit hei)—*inner heat.* A Traditional Chinese Medicine term, this condition is caused partly by dry, high-heat cooking.

以型補型 (yi xing bu xing; yi ying bou ying)—*eat the part to nourish the part.* Chinese people from some regions believe eating cooked animal brains will make them smarter, consuming an animal's feet will improve mobility, and so on.

美白 (mei bai; mei baak)—*white-beautifying.*

CHAPTER 11: CONFUSION

畫蛇添足 (hua she tian zu; waak se tim juk)—*drawing feet on snakes.* As unnecessary and unnatural as can be; purely wrong.

CHAPTER 12: HEALTH

忠言逆耳 (zhong yan ni er; jung yin yik yi)—*honest words prick the ears.* The truth hurts.

對牛彈琴 (dui niu tan qin; deui ngau taan kam)—*playing the zither to the cows.* Sending a good message to the wrong audience. They won't listen.

雞蛋裡挑骨頭 (ji dan li tiao gu tou; gai daan lieu tiu gwat tau)—*picking bones out of an egg.* A condition that doesn't exist. It is excessively demanding, worse than nitpicking. Chasing rainbows.

三寸金蓮 (san cun jin lian; saam chyun gam lin)—*a 3-inch lotus.* An attempt to look dainty and meet the social standard of beauty, such as binding the feet of girls in ancient China to look dainty.

事倍功半 (shi bei gong ban; si pui gung bun)—*doubling your efforts and halving your results.* Inefficient, waste of time.

事半功倍 (shi ban gong bei; si bun gung pui)—*only half the effort to see double the results.* Efficient, effortless beauty.

越 (yue; yuet)—*to excel and overcome.* My Chinese name. My Ba had high expectations of me. In turbulent times, to survive you must overcome.

CHAPTER 14: MY STORY

黑饃饃 (hei mo mo; haak mo mo)—*black buns.* Steam buns made from unprocessed grains.

洗臉洗腳洗屁股 (xi lian xi jiao xi pi gu; sai lim sai geuk sai pei gu)—*wash face, wash feet, wash bum bum.* Essentially, wash all the holes on your body.

缺一不可 (que yi b uke; kyut yat bat ho)—*won't have one without the other.* Can't live without either.

CHAPTER 15: YOUR WAY

三分鐘熱度 (san fen zhong re du; saam fan jung yit dou)—*3-minute passion.* A 3-minute, heated urge that doesn't last.

新屎坑三日香 (xin shi keng san ri xiang; san si haang saam yat heung)—*the new toilet even gets more poop.* Anything that's new will get more attention and use.

CONCLUSION

路遙知馬力, 日久見人心 (lu yao zhi ma li, ri jiu jian ren xin; lou you ji ma lik, yat gau gin yan sam)—*It takes distance to know a horse's strength, and it takes time to show a person's character.* Time will tell.

notes

1. 宇津木龍一Ryuichi Utsugi,「肌」の悩みがすべて消えるたった1つの方法 美肌には化粧水もクリームもいりません (Tokyo: Seishun Shuppansha Publishing Co., 2012).
2. 宇津木龍一Ryuichi Utsugi, 肌斷食, 譯. 婁愛蓮 (台灣 Taiwan: 方舟文化出版, 2013).
3. "Questionnaire Survey on Measures Against Skin Dryness," MyVoice Enquete Library, accessed August 18, 2020, https://myel.myvoice.jp/products/detail.php?product_id=12506.
4. "Survey on Sensitive Skin Prefectures and Generations with a Lot of Sensitive Skin?" Arouge Sensitive Skin Laboratory, accessed August 18, 2020, https://www.arouge.com/labo/basic/report171106.html.
5. "The Characteristics of Healthy Skin," Just About Skin, accessed August 25, 2020, http://www.justaboutskin.com/2016/01/what-is-healthy-skin/.
6. Selene K. Bantz, Zhou Zhu, and Tao Zheng, "The Atopic March: Progression from Atopic Dermatitis to Allergic Rhinitis and Asthma," *J Clin Cell Immunol* 5, no. 2 (April 2014): 202, Published online April 7, 2014, doi: 10.4172/2155-9899.1000202, https://www.ncbi.nlm.nih.gov/pmc/articles/PMC4240310/.
7. Sophie Nutten, "Atopic Dermatitis: Global Epidemiology and Risk Factors," *Annals of Nutrition and Metabolism* 66 Suppl. 1 (2015): 8–16.
8. Ramyani Gupta et al., "Time Trends in Allergic Disorders in the UK," *Thorax* 62.1 (2007): 91–96.
9. Joseph A. Odhiambo et al., "Global Variations in Prevalence of Eczema Symptoms in Children from ISAAC Phase Three," *Journal of Allergy and Clinical Immunology* 124.6 (2009): 1251–1258.

10　Sandy Skotnicki and Christopher Shulgan, "Do You Have Problem Skin?," in *Beyond Soap* (Canada: Penguin Random House, 2018), 12–15.

11　Jeremy Goldman, "Procter & Gamble Regains Its Title as Top Global Advertiser," eMarketer, accessed May 17, 2022, https://www.emarketer.com/content/procter-gamble-regains-its-title-top-global-advertiser.

12　Sandy Skotnicki and Christopher Shulgan, "The Cleanliness Obsession," in *Beyond Soap* (Canada: Penguin Random House, 2018), 21–37.

13　Geoffrey Jones, "Cleanliness and Civilization," in *Beauty Imagined* (UK: Oxford University Press, 2010), 75–77.

14　Sandy Skotnicki and Christopher Shulgan, "The Cleanliness Obsession," in *Beyond Soap* (Canada: Penguin Random House, 2018), 21–37.

15　Skotnicki and Shulgan, "The Cleanliness Obsession," 21–37.

16　SF Bloomfield et al., "Too Clean, or Not Too Clean: The Hygiene Hypothesis and Home Hygiene," *Clin Exp Allergy* 36, no. 4 (April 2006): 402–425, doi: 10.1111/j.1365-2222.2006.02463.x, https://www.ncbi.nlm.nih.gov/pmc/articles/PMC1448690/.

17　Karen Selick, "Coronavirus Crisis Reopens 150-Year-Old Controversy," accessed June 24, 2020, https://www.westernstandardonline.com/2020/04/selick-coronavirus-crisis-reopens-150-year-old-controversy/.

18　"The Microbe is Nothing…The Land Is Everything," French Institute of Human Sciences, accessed October 20, 2020, https://www.ifsh.fr/actualites/le-blog-ifsh/363-article-le-microbe-n-est-rien-le-terrain-est-tout.

19　Angel Corona, "Disease Eradication: What Does It Take to Wipe Out a Disease?" American Society for Microbiology, accessed October 20, 2020, https://asm.org/Articles/2020/March/Disease-Eradication-What-Does-It-Take-to-Wipe-out#:~:text=To%20date%2C%20the%20World%20Health,the%20rinderpest%20virus%20(RPV).

20　"The Top 10 Causes of Death," World Health Organization, accessed October 20, 2020, https://www.who.int/news-room/fact-sheets/detail/the-top-10-causes-of-death.

21　G.A.W. Rook, Charles Raison, and C.A. Lowry, "Microbial 'Old Friends,' Immunoregulation and Socioeconomic Status," *Clinical & Experimental Immunology* 177.1 (2014): 1–12.

22　S.F. Bloomfield, R. Standwell-Smith, and G.A. Rook, "The Hygiene Hypothesis and Its Implications for Home Hygiene, Lifestyle and Public Health: Summary," International Scientific Forum on Home Hygiene (2012).

23　Giulia Enders, "The Surprisingly Charming Science of Your Gut," TEDx, https://www.ted.com/talks/giulia_enders_the_surprisingly_charming_science_of_your_gut?language=en.

24 Geoffrey Jones, "Global Ambitions Meet Local Markets," in *Beauty Imagined* (United Kingdom: Oxford University Press, 2010), 211–222.
25 "Global Beauty and Personal Care Product Market Is Expected to Reach USD 756.63 Billion by 2026: Fior Markets," GlobeNewswire, accessed July 8, 2020, https://www.globenewswire.com/news-release/2020/01/24/1974743/0/en/Global-Beauty-and-Personal-Care-Product-Market-is-Expected-to-Reach-USD-756-63-Billion-by-2026-Fior-Markets.html.
26 "Revenue of the Leading 10 Beauty Manufacturers Worldwide in 2021," Statista, accessed February 28, 2022, https://www.statista.com/statistics/243871/revenue-of-the-leading-10-beauty-manufacturers-worldwide/.
27 Jeremy Goldman, "Procter & Gamble Regains Its Title as Top Global Advertiser," eMarketer, accessed May 17, 2022, https://www.emarketer.com/content/procter-gamble-regains-its-title-top-global-advertiser.
28 "How Much Is Your Face Worth?" About Face Skin Care, accessed July 8, 2020, https://aboutfaceskincare.com/blog/how-much-is-your-face-worth/.
29 Olay, accessed July 9, 2020, https://www.olay.ca/en-ca/skin-care-products/.
30 Andrew Jacono, "Quacks, Scams, and Botched Faces," in *The Park Avenue Face*, (Dallas: BenBella, 2019), 51–55.
31 "Cosmetics Overview," FDA U.S. Food & Drug Administration, accessed April 13, 2020, https://www.fda.gov/industry/regulated-products/cosmetics-overview.
32 "Alpha Hydroxy Acid Pioneers Honored," MDedge Dermatology, accessed May 17, 2022, https://www.mdedge.com/dermatology/article/18673/blog-alpha-hydroxy-acid-pioneers-honored.
33 M. Varinia Michalun and Joseph C. Dinardo, "Introduction," in *Milady Skin Care and Cosmetic Ingredients Dictionary*, 4th ed. (New York: Cengage Learning, 2015), 6.
34 J. L. St. Sauver et al., "Why Patients Visit Their Doctors: Assessing the Most Prevalent Conditions in a Defined American Population," *Mayo Clinic Proceedings* 88, no. 1 (January 2013): 56–67.
35 Ryuichi Utsugi, "How to Examine and Evaluate Skin Discoloration Using a Digital Microscope," The Japanese Society of Aesthetic Dermatology 19th Annual Meeting (Tokyo, Japan, August 23, 2001).
36 Ryuichi Utsugi, "A New Concept of Daily Skin Care Method: The Surprising Effects of Causes that Stopped Basic Cosmetic Entirely for Several Years," International Society of Aesthetic Plastic Surgery ISAPS (Kyoto, Japan, October 23, 2016).
37 Ryuichi Utsugi, "How to Examine and Evaluate Skin Discoloration Using a Digital Microscope," The Japanese Society of Aesthetic Dermatology 19th Annual Meeting (Tokyo, Japan, August 23, 2001).

38   Ryuichi Utsugi, "A New Concept of Daily Skin Care Method: The Surprising Effects of Causes that Stopped Basic Cosmetic Entirely for Several Years," International Society of Aesthetic Plastic Surgery ISAPS (Kyoto, Japan, October 23, 2016).

39   佐藤英明、宇津木龍一 Ryuichi Utsugi、山口麻子、矢沢慶史、塩谷信幸、内沼栄樹, "デジタルマイクロスコープによるくすみの診断法と一評価法について," 日本美容皮膚科学会会報 (2001.12, 23巻4号, 205頁).

40   工藤稚曜、宇津木龍一 Ryuichi Utsugi、佐藤英明、山口麻子、矢沢慶史, "ホームスキンケアシステムにおけるデジタルマイクロスコープの役割と有用性," 第19回日本美容皮膚科学会 (東京2001/08/23).

41   宇津木龍一 Ryuichi Utsugi、佐藤英明、山口麻子、矢沢慶史, "デジタルマイクロスコープによる肌診断支援ソフトの開発," 第19回日本美容皮膚科学会 (東京2001/08/23).

42   矢沢慶史、宇津木龍一Ryuichi Utsugi、佐藤英明、山口麻子, "グリコール酸、ビタミンC誘導体クリームによる毛孔の縮小効果," 第19回日本美容皮膚科学会 (東京2001/08/23).

43   M. Varinia Michalun and Joseph C. Dinardo, "Skin Anatomy & Physiology," in *Milady Skin Care and Cosmetic Ingredients Dictionary*, 4th ed. (New York: Cengage Learning, 2015), 15–17.

44   Wikipedia, s.v. "stratum corneum," accessed November 4, 2019, https://en.wikipedia.org/wiki/Stratum_corneum.

45   Wikipedia, s.v. "stratum corneum."

46   M. Varinia Michalun and Joseph C. Dinardo, "Skin Anatomy & Physiology," in *Milady Skin Care and Cosmetic Ingredients Dictionary*, 4th ed. (New York: Cengage Learning, 2015), 15–17.

47   Michalun and Dinardo, "Skin Anatomy & Physiology," 15–17.

48   Tim Taylor, "Integumentary System," Innerbody Research, accessed November 12, 2019, https://www.innerbody.com/anatomy/integumentary.

49   B. Alberts et al., "Epidermis and Its Renewal by Stem Cells," in *Molecular Biology of the Cell*, 4th ed. (New York: Garland Science, 2002), https://www.ncbi.nlm.nih.gov/books/NBK26865/.

50   M. Varinia Michalun and Joseph C. Dinardo, "Skin Anatomy & Physiology," in *Milady Skin Care and Cosmetic Ingredients Dictionary*, 4th ed. (New York: Cengage Learning, 2015), 15–17.

51   Ryuichi Utsugi 宇津木龍一, "Skin Structure 4: Natural Moisturizing Factor" in Skin Fasting肌斷食, trans. Ay-Lian Lou 譯. 婁愛蓮 (台灣 Taiwan: New Sino方舟文化出版, 2013), 70–75.

52   Tim Taylor, "Integumentary System," Innerbody Research, accessed November 12, 2019, https://www.innerbody.com/anatomy/integumentary.

53 Michael Specter, "Germs Are Us," *New Yorker*, accessed July 8, 2020, https://www.newyorker.com/magazine/2012/10/22/germs-are-us.
54 Elizabeth A. Grice and Julia A. Segre, "The Skin Microbiome," Nat Rev Microbiol. 9 no. 4 (April 2011): 244–253, doi: 10.1038/nrmicro2537, https://www.ncbi.nlm.nih.gov/pmc/articles/PMC3535073/.
55 Julia Benedetti, "Overview of Hypersensitivity and Reactive Skin Disorders," Merck Manuals, accessed September 27, 2020, https://www.merckmanuals.com/home/skin-disorders/hypersensitivity-and-inflammatory-skin-disorders/introduction-to-hypersensitivity-and-inflammatory-skin-disorders.
56 Kimberly Capone et al., "Diversity of the Human Skin Microbiome Early in Life," *Journal of Investigative Dermatology* 131.10 (2011): 2026–2032.
57 M. Varinia Michalun and Joseph C. Dinardo, "Skin Anatomy & Physiology," in *Milady Skin Care and Cosmetic Ingredients Dictionary*, 4th ed. (New York: Cengage Learning, 2015), 15–17.
58 Charlotte Cho, "The Magic of Exfoliation," in *The Little Book of Skin Care* (New York: HarperCollins), 51.
59 Robert B Zajonc, "Attitudinal Effects of Mere Exposure," *Journal of Personality and Social Psychology* 9 (1968): 1–27.
60 Julia Thomas, "What Is the Mere Exposure Effect?" BetterHelp, accessed October 13, 2020, https://www.betterhelp.com/advice/general/what-is-the-mere-exposure-effect/.
61 Leah Lawrence, "Cigarettes Were Once 'Physician' Tested, Approved," Healio, Hematology/Oncology, accessed November 8, 2021, https://www.healio.com/news/hematology-oncology/20120325/cigarettes-were-once-physician-tested-approved.
62 "President Nixon Signs Legislation Banning Cigarette Ads on TV and Radio," History, accessed November 8, 2021, https://www.history.com/this-day-in-history/nixon-signs-legislation-banning-cigarette-ads-on-tv-and-radio.
63 Sandy Skotnicki and Christopher Shulgan, "Do You Have Problem Skin?," in Beyond Soap (Canada: Penguin Random House, 2018), 12–15.
64 Kara Rogers, "Germ Theory," *Britannica Online*, accessed August 27, 2020, https://www.britannica.com/science/germ-theory.
65 Peter Attia, "Nutritional Biochemistry: #14 – Robert Lustig, M.D., M.S.L.: Fructose, Processed Food, NAFLD, and Changing the Food System," Peter Attia MD, accessed August 27, 2020, https://peterattiamd.com/roblustig/.
66 Wikipedia, s.v. "L'Oréal," accessed March 21, 2020, https://en.wikipedia.org/wiki/L%27Or%C3%A9al.
67 Steve Milano, "What Is Vertical Segmentation?," Chron, accessed February 26, 2022, https://smallbusiness.chron.com/vertical-segmentation-61866.html.

68 David Sinclair, *Lifespan: Why We Age—and Why We Don't Have To* (US: Atria Books, 2019).
69 *Britannica Online*, s.v. "sebaceous gland," accessed November 20, 2021, https://www.britannica.com/science/sebaceous-gland.
70 Yashoda, "Difference Between Sebaceous and Sweat Glands," Difference Between, accessed November 20, 2021, https://www.differencebetween.com/difference-between-sebaceous-and-vs-sweat-glands/.
71 Wikipedia, s.v. "surfactant," accessed November 14, 2019, https://en.wikipedia.org/wiki/Surfactant.
72 Yan Zheng and Xuebing Xu, "Hydrophilic-Lipophilic Balance," ScienceDirect, accessed October 26, 2020, https://www.sciencedirect.com/topics/agricultural-and-biological-sciences/hydrophilic-lipophilic-balance.
73 Morgan B. Murphrey, Julia H. Miao, and Patrick M. Zito, "Histology, Stratum Corneum," National Library of Medicine, https://www.ncbi.nlm.nih.gov/books/NBK513299/.
74 Whitney Bowe and Kristin Loberg, "Nature's Hidden Secret to Great Skin," in *The Beauty of Dirty Skin* (New York: Little, Brown and Company, 2018), 32.
75 Jixin Zhong and Guixiu Shi, "Editorial: Regulation of Inflammation in Chronic Disease," Front. *Immunol.* 12 (April 2019), https://doi.org/10.3389/fimmu.2019.00737, https://www.frontiersin.org/articles/10.3389/fimmu.2019.00737/full.
76 Roma Pahwa, Amandeep Goyal, and Ishwarlal Jialal, "Chronic Inflammation," National Library of Medicine, https://www.ncbi.nlm.nih.gov/books/NBK493173/.
77 "How Your Body Repairs Cuts," Ask A Biologist, Arizona State University, accessed October 10, 2020, https://askabiologist.asu.edu/wound-healing.
78 "Understanding and Managing Chronic Inflammation," Healthline, accessed October 16, 2020, https://www.healthline.com/health/chronic-inflammation.
79 "Understanding and Managing Chronic Inflammation," Healthline.
80 Paula Begoun, "Skin's Enemy: Irritation and Inflammation," in *The Original Beauty Bible*, 3rd ed. (Washington: Beginning Press, 2009), 77.
81 "Inflammation and Auto-Inflammation," SickKids, AboutKidsHealth, accessed December 6, 2020, https://www.aboutkidshealth.ca/Article?contentid=926&language=English.
82 Sandy Skotnicki and Christopher Shulgan, "Damaging Our Body's Natural Armour," in *Beyond Soap* (Canada: Penguin Random House, 2018), 46–47.
83 "Eczema Statistics," MG217, accessed February 19, 2022, https://mg217.com/your-eczema/statistics/.
84 Sophie Nutten, "Atopic Dermatitis: Global Epidemiology and Risk Factors," *Annals of Nutrition and Metabolism* 66 Suppl. 1 (2015): 8–16.

85   Sandy Skotnicki and Christopher Shulgan, "Introduction," in *Beyond Soap* (Canada: Penguin Random House, 2018), 1–3.
86   SF Bloomfield et al., "Too Clean, or Not Too Clean: The Hygiene Hypothesis and Home Hygiene," *Clin Exp Allergy* 36, no. 4 (April 2006): 402–425, doi: 10.1111/j.1365-2222.2006.02463.x, https://www.ncbi.nlm.nih.gov/pmc/articles/PMC1448690/.
87   Sandy Skotnicki and Christopher Shulgan, "Do You Have Problem Skin?," in *Beyond Soap* (Canada: Penguin Random House, 2018), 12–15.
88   A. K. DeGruttola et al., "Current Understanding of Dysbiosis in Disease in Human and Animal Models," *Inflammatory Bowel Disease* 22, no. 5 (May 2016): 1137–50.
89   J. P. McFadden, "The Great Atopic Disease Epidemic: Does Chemical Exposure Play a Role?" *British Journal of Dermatology* 166.6 (2012): 1156–1157.
90   S. K. Bantz, Z. Zhu, and T. Zheng, "The Atopic March: Progression from Atopic Dermatitis to Allergic Rhinitis and Asthma," *Journal of Clinical and Cellular Immunology* 5.2 (2014): 202.
91   Andrea Sherriff, J. Golding, and Alspac Study Team, "Hygiene Levels in a Contemporary Population Cohort Are Associated with Wheezing and Atopic Eczema in Preschool Infants," *Archives of Disease in Childhood* 87.1 (2002): 26–29, https://pubmed.ncbi.nlm.nih.gov/12089117/.
92   "Skin Care Market in the U.S.," Statista, accessed April 27, 2020, https://www.statista.com/topics/4517/us-skin-care-market/.
93   Sandy Skotnicki and Christopher Shulgan, "Introduction," in *Beyond Soap* (Canada: Penguin Random House, 2018), 1–3.
94   J. L. St. Sauver et al., "Why Patients Visit Their Doctors: Assessing the Most Prevalent Conditions in a Defined American Population," *Mayo Clinic Proceedings* 88, no. 1 (January 2013): 56–67.
95   "How Often Do Children Need to Take a Bath?" American Academy of Dermatology, September 12, 2016, https://www.aad.org/public/everyday-care/skin-care-basics/care/child-bathing#:~:text=Children%20ages%206%20to%2011,once%20or%20twice%20a%20week.
96   Andrew Jacono, "Begin with the Skin," in *The Park Avenue Face* (Dallas: BenBella, 2019), 74.
97   "Routine Childbirth Episiotomies Do More Harm than Good," *Globe and Mail*, accessed December 16, 2020, https://www.theglobeandmail.com/life/routine-childbirth-episiotomies-do-more-harm-than-good/article1037229/.
98   K. Bhate and H. C. Williams, "Epidemiology of Acne Vulgaris," *The British Journal of Dermatology* 168 (2013): 474–485.
99   Bhate and Williams, "Epidemiology of Acne Vulgaris," 474–485.
100 K. Bhate and H. C. Williams, "Epidemiology of Acne Vulgaris," 474–485.

101 Andrew Jacono, "Quacks, Scams, and Botched Faces," in *The Park Avenue Face* (Dallas: BenBella, 2019), 51–55.
102 Peter Attia, "#188 – AMA #30: How to Read and Understand Scientific Studies," Peter Attia MD, https://peterattiamd.com/ama30/.
103 "Skin Care Market in the U.S.," Statista, accessed April 27, 2020, https://www.statista.com/topics/4517/us-skin-care-market/.
104 "Your Questions Answered," Vaseline, accessed August 16, 2021, https://www.vaseline.com/in/en/contact-us/faq.html.
105 "Bar Soap's Bad Rap. What Millennials Got Wrong," Island Thyme Soap, accessed October 1, 2021, https://islandthymesoap.com/blogs/latest/bar-soaps-bad-rap.
106 J. E. Heinze and F. Yackovich, "Washing with Contaminated Bar Soap is Unlikely to Transfer Bacteria," *Epidemiol Infect.* 101, no. 1 (August 1988): 135–142, doi: 10.1017/s0950268800029290, https://www.ncbi.nlm.nih.gov/pmc/articles/PMC2249330/.
107 "What is Natural Soap Made Of?" Seatree, accessed October 21, 2021, https://www.seatree.org.uk/blog/what-is-natural-soap-made-of/.
108 "How Does Soap Work?" Hackensack Meridian Health, accessed October 29, 2021, https://www.hackensackmeridianhealth.org/HealthU/2020/08/11/how-does-soap-work/.
109 "Formulations Regular Soaps Combars And Syndets," GUWS Medical, accessed October 29, 2021, https://www.guwsmedical.info/contact-dermatitis/formulations-regular-soaps-combars-and-syndets.html.
110 Ehrhardt Proksch, "Buffering Capacity," Curr Probl Dermatology 54 (2018):11–18, doi: 10.1159/000489513, Epub August 21, 2018, https://pubmed.ncbi.nlm.nih.gov/30130768/.
111 "Your Skin," KidsHealth, accessed June 24, 2020, https://kidshealth.org/en/kids/skin.html.
112 Yana Mandeville, "Jane Fonda, Beauty Of Audacity," HealthyLiving, accessed June 24, 2020, https://www.healthylivingmagazine.us/Articles/10479/.
113 J. Lewis et al., "Epidermis and Its Renewal by Stem Cells," in *Molecular Biology of the Cell.* 4th edition, (New York: Garland Science; 2002), https://www.ncbi.nlm.nih.gov/books/NBK26865/.
114 Agata Dabrowska and Susan Thaul, "How FDA Approves Drugs and Regulates Their Safety and Effectiveness," Congressional Research Service, May 8, 2018, https://fas.org/sgp/crs/misc/R41983.pdf.
115 "Consulting Canadians on the Regulation of Self-Care Products in Canada," Government of Canada, accessed April 21, 2020, https://www.canada.ca/en/health-canada/programs/consultation-regulation-self-care-products/consulting-canadians-regulation-self-care-products-canada.html.

116 "Consulting Canadians on the Regulation of Self-Care Products in Canada," accessed April 21, 2020.
117 R Hauser and A Calafat, "Phthalates and Human Health," *Occup Environ Med.* 62, no. 11 (November 2005): 806–818, doi: 10.1136/oem.2004.017590, https://www.ncbi.nlm.nih.gov/pmc/articles/PMC1740925/.
118 Christy L. De Vader and Paxson Barker, "Fragrance in the Workplace Is the New Second-Hand Smoke," Proceedings of ASBBS 16, no. 1, ASBBS Annual Conference: Las Vegas, February 2009, https://www.national-toxic-encephalopathy-foundation.org/fragsmoke.pdf.
119 Adi Pinkas, Cinara Ludvig Gonçalves and Michael Aschner, "Neurotoxicity of Fragrance Compounds: A Review," *Environ Res* 158 (October 2017): 342–349, doi: 10.1016/j.envres.2017.06.035. Epub 2017 Jul 3, https://www.ncbi.nlm.nih.gov/pubmed/28683407.
120 Justin Marchegiani, "Fragrance: The New Secondhand Smoke," Just in Health, accessed November 16, 2021, https://justinhealth.com/fragrance-the-new-secondhand-smoke/.
121 M. Varinia Michalun and Joseph C. Dinardo, "How Products Work," in *Milady Skin Care and Cosmetic Ingredients Dictionary*, 4th ed. (New York: Cengage Learning, 2015), 45–63.
122 Carsten R. Hamann et al., "Is There a Risk Using Hypoallergenic Cosmetic Pediatric Products in the United States?" *Journal of Allergy and Clinical Immunology* 135.4 (2015): 1070–1071.
123 "Projected Market Value of Organic Personal Care Worldwide from 2018 to 2025," Statista, https://www.statista.com/statistics/943705/organic-personal-care-market-value-worldwide/.
124 Sandy Skotnicki and Christopher Shulgan, "Minimalist Skincare," in *Beyond Soap* (Canada: Penguin Random House, 2018), 230–237.
125 Peter Attia, "#188—AMA #30: How to Read and Understand Scientific Studies." Peter Attia MD, https://peterattiamd.com/ama30/.
126 Peter Attia, "#188—AMA #30: How to Read and Understand Scientific Studies."
127 Peter Attia, "#188—AMA #30: How to Read and Understand Scientific Studies."
128 "Audrey Hepburn Smoking Facts," accessed July 20, 2021, https://www.everythingaudrey.com/audrey-hepburn-smoking-facts-and-images/.
129 "Tobacco Use in Racial and Ethnic Populations," American Lung Association, accessed July 20, 2020, https://www.lung.org/quit-smoking/smoking-facts/impact-of-tobacco-use/tobacco-use-racial-and-ethnic.
130 Albert L. Hermalin and Deborah Lowry, "The Age Prevalence of Smoking Among Chinese Women: A Case of Arrested Diffusion?," Population Studies Center Research Report, October 2010, University of Michigan, Institute for Social Research, https://www.psc.isr.umich.edu/pubs/pdf/rr10-718.pdf.

131 "Photoaging: What You Need to Know About the Other Kind of Aging," Skin Cancer Foundation, accessed July 14, 2021, https://www.skincancer.org/blog/photoaging-what-you-need-to-know/.

132 Sandy Skotnicki and Christopher Shulgan, "Minimalist Skincare," in Beyond Soap (Canada: Penguin Random House, 2018), 230–237.

133 Charlotte Cho, "Sunscreen: The Most Important Word in Skin Care," in *The Little Book of Skin Care* (New York: HarperCollins, November 2015), 90–91.

134 Whitney Bowe and Kristin Loberg, "Feed Your Face," in *The Beauty of Dirty Skin* (New York: Little, Brown and Company, 2018), 123–126.

135 Whitney Bowe, S. S. Joshi, and A. R. Shalita, "Diet and Acne," *Journal of the American Academy of Dermatology* 63, no. 1 (July 2010): 124–41.

136 Whitney Bowe and Kristin Loberg, "Introduction," in *The Beauty of Dirty Skin* (New York: Little, Brown and Company, 2018), 13.

137 Rajani Katta and Samir Desai, "Diet and Dermatology: The Role of Dietary Intervention in Skin Disease," *The Journal of Clinical and Aesthetic Dermatology* 7.7 (2014): 46.

138 Whitney Bowe and Kristin Loberg, "Feed Your Face," in *The Beauty of Dirty Skin* (New York: Little, Brown and Company, 2018), 123–126.

139 J. Uribarri et al., "Diet-Derived Advanced Glycation End Products Are Major Contributors to the Body's AGE Pool and Induce Inflammation in Healthy Subjects," *Annals of the New York Academy of Sciences* 1043 (2005): 461–466.

140 "Unhappy Meals," *New York Times Magazine*, accessed July 15, 2021, https://www.nytimes.com/2007/01/28/magazine/28nutritionism.t.html.

141 "Unhappy Meals," *New York Times Magazine*.

142 "Unhappy Meals," *New York Times Magazine*.

143 "Why the Fountain of Youth Might Taste Very Salty," Daily News, McMaster University, accessed November 28, 2021, https://dailynews.mcmaster.ca/articles/why-the-fountain-of-youth-might-taste-very-salty/.

144 Anke Huls et al., "Traffic-Related Air Pollution Contributes to Development of Facial Lentigines: Further Epidemiological Evidence from Caucasians and Asians," *Journal of Investigative Dermatology* 136.5 (2016): 1053–1056.

145 Damian Carrington, "Air Pollution Causes Wrinkles and Premature Ageing, New Research Shows," *Guardian*, July 15, 2016, https://www.theguardian.com/environment/2016/jul/15/air-pollution-causes-wrinkles-and-premature-ageing-new-research-shows.

146 J.P. Majra, "Air Quality in Rural Areas," in Nicolas Mazzeo, ed. *Chemistry, Emission Control, Radioactive Pollution and Indoor Air Quality* (London: IntechOpen, 2011), 10.5772/1030, https://www.intechopen.com/chapters/16341.

147 Paul Tullis, "The Man Who Can Map the Chemicals All Over Your Body," *Nature* 534.7606 (2016): 170–172.

148 Amina Bouslimani et al., "Molecular Cartography of the Human Skin Surface in 3D," *Proceedings of the National Academy of Sciences* 112.17 (2015): E2120–E2129.
149 Elena Figuero et al., "Mechanical and Chemical Plaque Control in the Simultaneous Management of Gingivitis and Caries: a Systematic Review," Journal of Clin Periodontol 44 Suppl 18 (March 2017): S116–S134, doi: 10.1111/jcpe.12674, https://pubmed.ncbi.nlm.nih.gov/28266113/.
150 Wikipedia, s.v. "precautionary principle," accessed July 6, 2020, https://en.wikipedia.org/wiki/Precautionary_principle.
151 "Compliance Bias," Catalogue of Bias, Accessed July 7, 2020, https://catalogofbias.org/biases/compliance-bias/.
152 Peter Attia, "Studying Studies: Part I—Relative Risk vs. Absolute Risk," Peter Attia MD, accessed November 28, 2021, https://peterattiamd.com/ns001/.
153 Yana Mandeville, "Jane Fonda, Beauty Of Audacity," HealthyLiving, accessed June 24, 2020, https://www.healthylivingmagazine.us/Articles/10479/.
154 "The Transtheoretical Model (Stages of Change)," Behavioral Change Models, accessed November 28, 2021, https://sphweb.bumc.bu.edu/otlt/mph-modules/sb/behavioralchangetheories/behavioralchangetheories6.html.
155 "Sugar: The Bitter Truth," YouTube, University of California Television (UCTV), https://www.youtube.com/watch?v=dBnniua6-oM.
156 "What It's Like to Quit Smoking," U.S. Food and Drug Administration, accessed August 5, 2021, https://www.fda.gov/tobacco-products/health-information/quitting-smoking-closer-every-attempt.
157 Peter Attia, "Qualy #29—Fasting as a Powerful Drug in the Toolbox of Medicine," Peter Attia MD, accessed August 16, 2021, https://peterattiamd.com/qualy-29-fasting-as-a-powerful-drug-in-the-toolbox/.
158 Cal Newport, *Deep Work: Rules for Focused Success in a Distracted World* (New York: Grand Central Publishing, 2016).
159 Yuval Noah Harari, "There is No Justice in History," in *Sapiens: A Brief History of Humankind* (Canada: Signal, 2014), 145.
160 Wikipedia, s.v. "Cultural Revolution," accessed October 10, 2021, https://en.wikipedia.org/wiki/Cultural_Revolution.
161 Valerie Strauss and Daniel Southerl, "How Many Died? New Evidence Suggests Far Higher Numbers for the Victims of Mao Zedong's Era," *Washington Post*, accessed October 10, 2021, https://www.washingtonpost.com/archive/politics/1994/07/17/how-many-died-new-evidence-suggests-far-higher-numbers-for-the-victims-of-mao-zedongs-era/01044df5-03dd-49f4-a453-a033c5287bce/.
162 Michael Pollan, *In Defense of Food: An Eater's Manifesto* (New York: Penguin Press, 2008).

163 "A Brief History of Skincare Through the Ages," INB Medical, accessed May 2, 2022, https://www.inbmedical.com/the-evolving-role-of-skincare.

164 Wikipedia, s.v. "Cosmetics in Korea," accessed September 28, 2020, https://en.wikipedia.org/wiki/Cosmetics_in_Korea.

about the authors

ERIN YUET TJAM—
THE BEAUTY-OBSESSED SCIENTIST

Erin's vanity is known to all her friends, and her six kids—but so is her persistent quest for knowledge and improvement.

Not very many people would graduate top of her year with scholarships and awards (BSc from McGill), and not work a single day in the field. It was just because she found out her food scientist job required her to wear a lab coat and hair net—an affront to her personal style!

How often does a young mom of a toddler dare to rock the boat of a cushy speech language pathologist job (MHSc from Toronto) to compete for a Health Canada research grant? Winning it would mean a fully funded doctoral degree and living expenses, but a complicated life with part-time work, part-time study, and full-time motherhood. Erin won the grant, completed her PhD in less than three years, and defended before delivery—her thesis was born a few days before her second son. Finishing a PhD in two years and nine months was a record completion time even for full-time students at the University of Waterloo. Her thesis passed with no revisions—but whether it was because she did a fine job or her all-male committee was scared her baby would pop out remains a closely guarded secret.

Twelve years of education seemed like a breeze compared to working in the real world and being a career mom. After her PhD in Health Studies, Dr. Tjam joined a pharmaceutical research firm in Toronto, and she became a mother again in less than two years. Life was madness with three sporty and musical boys. Her busy family brought her work back to Waterloo, where she was the Director of Research at St. Mary's General Hospital and Senior Research Associate at St. Joseph's Healthcare for nearly 12 years. Concurrently, Dr. Tjam held adjunct professor and health researcher positions with UW, as well as honorary professorships with several universities in China. Throughout her research career, Dr. Tjam has published in numerous peer-reviewed journals and has been awarded over $7.5 million in research grants.

The working world was challenging, but running her own business was a lot more high-stakes and rewarding. Erin's entrepreneurial endeavors began when David Johnston, the previous Governor General of Canada, appointed her as his special advisor when he was the President of UW. Erin founded a joint venture with UW in international training for senior executives. This expanded into hospitality real estate, where Erin established operational systems so her dependable staff could run the business while she focused on other developments.

Erin has lived in many places in China, Hong Kong, and Canada, and is bilingual and bicultural. She and her husband, Bruce, are parents to six wonderful grown children. Together, with grandparents Gong Gong and Po Po, Erin and Bruce have managed a vibrant household of 10 people living under the same roof for over a decade. Now that the nest is getting smaller, Erin is devoting her time to learning, deepening her relationships, and being healthy.

She got back to downhill skiing 4 years ago at 53, initially to please her skier husband, but fell in love with the sport and became insanely devoted to the ideal of being a *good-looking* skier. She skis with Bruce, their kids, and friends in the big mountains of Western Canada, Colorado, Europe, and Japan many weeks a season, and she races on tiny local hills. The whole point is so she can ski gracefully enough to deserve fab ski suits. Erin practices yoga regularly under the coaching of an Olympic swimmer turned yogi, and she cycles long distances with Bruce at home and on trips. Recently, Erin fell in love, alongside Bruce, with playing pickleball. They play 6.5 times a week! All so she can eat to her heart's desire, have a good figure, and live long. She and Bruce also enjoy fasting, raising chickens and ducks, fishing in their pond, gardening, cooking, and hosting parties at their country home.

For over 40 years, Erin read, researched, and experimented about anything she could find on skin. So, becoming a published author on a public health book dressed up as beauty is a dream come true for this girly girl and scientist. Publishing a "skin-deep" book beats writing scientific articles that are lucky to get 50 readers 😊. Erin would be happy if she could just get all her kids and future grandkids to do *Skin Sobering*.

RYUICHI UTSUGI— THE ANTI-AGING DOCTOR

Dr. Utsugi is a board-certified plastic surgeon who founded the Division of Plastic & Aesthetic Surgery and the Aesthetic Medicine Center at Kitasato University School of Medicine, where he worked for 27 years. His specialties were maxillofacial and rejuvenation surgery and dermatology. As the chief plastic surgeon of the critical care center, he treated patients with burns daily. He found that except for pure petroleum jelly, no other topical compounds were ever used to treat burns. Creams and lotions of all kinds prevented wounds from healing.

Dr. Utsugi's expertise in the treatment of burns helped him develop a skin care method that is truly good for the skin and for the pocket. Besides being a physician, Dr. Utsugi was also an expert advisor to cosmetic companies and aesthetic salons. He had his own line of skincare products before he discovered the harms these products do to the skin.

For 17 years, he focused on the development of rejuvenation surgery for the aged face. However, he found that older faces do not look young with surgery alone. They also need to have beautiful and youthful-looking skin. From his work with thousands of patients, Dr. Utsugi discovered that if they did not apply skincare products before and after surgery, their skin would be hydrated, young, and smooth. Not surprisingly, as soon as the patient began using skincare products, their natural skin felt drier and looked worse. This happened in every case. Clinical data in the thousands convinced Dr. Utsugi that the best form of skin care, for patients and people in general, is *Skin Sobering*. He presented the findings to and published them in many scientific venues.

Ryuichi is also a meticulous artist. His favorite hobby is carving Noh masks, which are full facial masks worn in classical Japanese dance-drama. This hobby alongside his profession gave him a unique talent for judging human faces. On the physical side, Ryuichi skis and loves martial arts, especially Kendo and Shorinji Kempo, in which he has achieved black belt status. Ryuichi is expanding his love of martial arts to MMA, specifically Brazilian Jiu-Jitsu, and he is determined to reach his personal best after he retires.

Underneath this "tough man kung fu fighting" hard shell, Ryuichi is a softy at heart. He is devoted to Noriko, his wife of 31 years, and to his only daughter. Ryuichi frequently speaks lovingly of his wife, Noriko. In addition to being an accomplished educator, author, and illustrator, Noriko has always been a very beautiful woman. Today, she is cool, uncomplicated, and even more attractive. "Noriko is the woman I still yearn for, inside and out."

Dr. Utsugi is a "physician of conscience 有良知的醫生" who saved our skin—this is heartfelt praise from his Asian readers. We are fortunate to have doctors like him, especially when too many medical professionals are caught between securing profits versus serving patients.

professional achievements

Dr. Erin Yuet Tjam, PhD, has had a rich career over the last thirty years. She has been a health educator, adjunct professor, entrepreneur, and Special Advisor to the President at the University of Waterloo. She was also Director of Research at St. Mary's General Hospital and Health Researcher at St. Joseph's Health Care System, in Ontario, Canada. Erin established two successful businesses while managing a vibrant household of six kids and two grandparents. Now that the kids are grown and the businesses are self-sufficient, she devotes her time to researching and writing about health and beauty. Erin has been obsessed with skin for over four decades.

Dr. Ryuichi Utsugi, MD, is a specialist in anti-aging and skin health, and a board-certified plastic surgeon for over forty years. He founded the Aesthetic Medicine Center of the Research Institute of Kitasato University Hospital and is the Director of Clinic UTSUGIryu in Tokyo, Japan. He was an expert advisor to skincare companies and had his own line of skincare products before he discovered what they do to the skin. He presented and published this research in conferences, scientific papers, medical textbooks, and skin health books. One of his books, translated in Chinese as *Skin Fasting*, remains popular across Asia a decade after publication in Japan.

Printed in Great Britain
by Amazon